WM845DOW

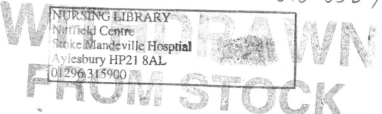
ersity o
rdshir

Down Syndrome:
A Review of Current Knowledge

?

3

Down Syndrome: A Review of Current Knowledge

EDITED BY
Jean A Rondal, PhD (Psy), D Ling
Juan Perera DPsy
and
Lynn Nadel PhD (Psy)

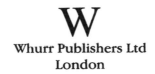

Whurr Publishers Ltd
London

© 1999 Whurr Publishers Ltd
First published 1999 by Whurr Publishers Ltd
19b Compton Terrace, London N1 2UN, England

British Library Cataloguing-in-Publication Data
A catalogue record for this book is available from the British Library.

ISBN 1 86156 062 1

Printed and bound in Great Britain by Athenæum Press Ltd, Gateshead, Tyne & Wear.

Contents

Acknowledgements
The VI World Congress on
Down Syndrome

This book is a direct product of the VI World Congress on Down Syndrome held in Madrid, Spain, from 23 to 26 October 1997, on the theme: *Down syndrome: when dreams come true*. As President of the Congress, it is my pleasure to acknowledge the contributions of a number of individual persons and institutions without whose help the Congress would not have been possible. I wish to thank particularly Her Majesty Doña Sophia, Queen of Spain, President of the Honor Committee; Professor-Dr Jean A Rondal, Vice-President of the Congress and President of the European Down Syndrome Association; Professor Alberto Rasore-Quartino, Secretary of the Congress; the Federación Española de Instituciones para el Síndrome de Down (FEISD); The European Down Syndrome Association (EDSA); and the International Down Syndrome Federation (IDSF), as coorganizing partners. I am grateful to the United Nations Educational, Scientific, and Cultural Organization (UNESCO); the Ministerio Español de Trabajo y Asuntos Sociales; the Ministerio Español de Sanidad y Consumo; the Ministerio Español de Educación y Cultura; the Universidad Complutense de Madrid; the Ayuntamiento de Madrid, Convention Bureau; as well as to Viajes Iberia Congress for their special collaboration.

I also wish to acknowledge the sponsorship of various entities: the Asociación Síndrome de Down de Baleares (ASNIMO); the Instituto Español de Migraciones y Servicios Sociales (IMSESO); the Real Patronato de Prevención y de Atención a Personas con Minusvalia; the Fundación ONCE para la Cooperación e Integración Social de Personas con Minusvalias; the Gabinete LLOS; the Mutualidad de Previsión Social; the Cadena SOL MELIÀ; the Fundación Inocente; Grespania; Iberia Lineas Aéreas de España; Telefónica; and MRW.

Lastly, I should like to express a warm thank you to the following persons for generously dispensing their time and efforts in the preparation and during the time of the congress: D Manuel Ramiro; Doña Carmen

Crespo; D José Botella; D Antonio de la Torra; D Andrés Martinez; Doña
Marta Sutil; and the Asociación Síndrome de Down de Madrid.

Juan Perera
President of the VI World Congress on Down Syndrome
President of the Federación Española de Instituciones para el Síndrome
de Down
Former President of the Scientific Committee of the European Down
Syndrome Association

Contributors

Marjorie Beeghly Child Development Unit, Children's Hospital and Harvard University, Boston, USA

Lars-Åke Berglund Handitek Foundation, Borlange, Sweden

Anders Bond Handitek Foundation, Borlange, Sweden

Sue Buckley The Sarah Duffen Centre & Department of Psychology, University of Portsmouth, Southsea, UK

Charles J Epstein Department of Pediatrics, University of California, San Francisco, USA

David W Evans Department of Psychology, University of New Orleans, New Orleans, USA

Alberto Fortuny Obstetrics and Gynaecology Service, University of Barcelona Hospital, Barcelona, Spain

Carmen García Pastor Department of Didactics and School Organization, Faculty of Sciences of Education, University of Seville, Seville, Spain.

F Lee Gray Department of Psychology, University of New Orleans, New Orleans, USA

Michael J Guralnick Human Development Center, University of Washington, Seattle, USA

Robert Hodapp Graduate School of Education and Information, University of California, Los Angeles, USA

Dianne M McBrien Division of Developmental Disabilities, Department of Pediatrics, University of Iowa Hospitals and Clinics, Iowa City, USA

Enrico Montobbio Centre for the Study of the Integration of Disabled People, Genova, Italy

Lynn Nadel Department of Psychology, University of Arizona, Tucson, USA

Juan Perera Centre Prince of Asturias and University of the Balearic Islands, Palma de Mallorca, Spain

Mario C Peterson Division of Developmental Disabilities, Department of Pediatrics, University of Iowa Hospitals and Clinics, Iowa City, USA

Siegfried M Pueschel Rhode Island Hospital Child Development Center and Brown University Department of Pediatrics, Rhode Island, USA

Alberto Rasore-Quartino Department of Neonatology, Galliera Hospitals, Genova, Italy

Jean A Rondal Psycholinguistic Laboratory, University of Liège, Liège, Belgium

John E Rynders Department of Educational Psychology, University of Minnesota, Minneapolis, USA

Siraj U Siddiqi Division of Developmental Disabilities, Department of Pediatrics, University of Iowa Hospitals and Clinics, Iowa City, USA

Wayne Silverman Institute for Basic Research in Developmental Disabilities, Staten Island, New York, USA

Pierre-Marie Sinet Faculty of Medicine, Necker Hospital for Sick Children, Paris, France

Don C Van Dyke Division of Developmental Disabilities, Department of Pediatrics, University of Iowa Hospitals and Clinics, Iowa City, USA

Jan-Erik Wänn Handitek Foundation, Borlange, Sweden

Henryk Wisniewski Institute for Basic Research in Developmental Disabilities, Staten Island, New York, USA

PART 1
INTRODUCTION

Chapter 1
The Person with Down Syndrome

SIEGFRIED M. PUESCHEL

From ancient history up to the present time, every society has been confronted with the problem of what to do with those who are unable to meet the demands and expectations of their respective cultures. There were times when mentally handicapped persons were believed to be possessed with evil spirits and when they were viewed as a burden to civilization. There were times when they were shunned, exploited, and persecuted. There were also periods in history when persons with handicapping conditions were objects of amusement or when they were regarded as supernatural beings. Here reverence - there persecution - all routed in superstition. Less often did individuals with mental retardation, including those with Down syndrome, receive kind treatment and rarely were they protected from a cruel environment and looked upon as individuals with rights.

It was only during the past century, when science superseded sorcery, that society gradually changed its attitude toward persons with developmental disabilities. In particular, significant progress has been made during the past few decades. Parents of children with mental retardation including those with Down syndrome requested that their children be given the same rights and opportunities that were available to nonhandicapped children and subsequently new approaches in the care, treatment, and education of persons with mental retardation evolved. During the past decades, scientific advances have been made not only in the biomedical arena but also in the field of behavioural science.

Most importantly, positive changes have taken place in the humanitarian approach to the care of persons with developmental disabilities including those with Down syndrome. Today we know that persons with mental retardation have an intrinsic value of humanity. We also know that they can contribute to society and perform tasks which previously were never expected of them.

Currently we realize that persons with Down syndrome are individuals in their own right in spite of their limited capacity for academic achievement. Individuals with Down syndrome let us know that they are able to learn, that they can have fun, be responsible, dependable, and can work hard. Persons with Down syndrome have feelings like other human beings and they have ups and downs. They will be happy when things go well, and they will be sad when they are offended or looked upon as second-class citizens. Persons with Down syndrome demonstrate that they do not have to be segregated, institutionalized, and shunned away, but can be active participants in community life. Displaying a diversity of human abilities and functions, persons with Down syndrome make us aware of the fact that looking upon them with respect and dignity is of utmost importance.

Persons with Down syndrome teach us that using quality as a measure of relationship brings a dimension that quantity cannot match. Often persons with Down syndrome will accept you and love you for who you are. Really knowing a person with Down syndrome will make your life richer and you will feel a deep sense of appreciation for having had the opportunity to meet this person in real life.

The value of persons with Down syndrome is intrinsically rooted in their humanity and in their uniqueness as human beings. If individuals with Down syndrome are considered to be human, and thus have the intrinsic value and the rights of a human being, they can reach a point of significant fulfilment of their limited potentialities.

When it comes to life there are no limits. There is a tremendous potential within each person with Down syndrome, a potential that can be reached if we are sincere in providing all of them with optimal medical, educational, recreational, and vocational services, and if we are dedicated to enhancing the fullness of life of every person with Down syndrome.

In recent years, there has been a profound surge of awareness of the dignity and human rights of people with developmental disabilities including those with Down syndrome. Inherent in the presently prevailing philosophy is the realization that nobody is perfect, that we all have our own personalities, our own unique abilities, and our own strengths and weaknesses. We can appreciate a child's individual beauty, whatever it is, no matter how seriously handicapped that child may be. If one believes that human life is infinite in value, then one must believe that the sanctity of life is bound to be unaffected by either mental or physical defects. We must preserve our humanity and our human values in a world whose forces, pressures, and seductions tell us to believe in technology and technological solutions.

All human behaviour takes place in an ethical context based on values. These values determine what we believe to be right and wrong. We must be clear about what our values are and how these values influence our behaviour. For professionals in the field of mental retardation, the basic thrust should be recognition of the dignity and worth of people with Down syndrome. The primary goal should be to improve the quality of their lives as much as possible. Service to humanity must rank higher than any other personal gratification in professional life. It takes courage to push yourself to places you have never been, to test your limits, and to break through barriers.

We have to foster optimal well being of persons with Down syndrome in all areas of human functioning. For, if provided with appropriate health care, excellent education and if offered meaningful vocational experiences, individuals with Down syndrome can live a more fulfilling life. A humane society should demonstrate its concerns by providing the emotional, financial, educational and other supports needed by families courageously refusing to let the quality overshadow equality.

In spite of the significant progress that has been made in the field of developmental disabilities during the past decades, the humaneness of all persons with Down syndrome is still not fully established. There are still people who view individuals with Down syndrome as subhuman. These older images are deeply imbedded in the public consciousness and in the residual of old customs and laws. Some people still cling to an antiquated view which is primarily based on false assumptions about persons with Down syndrome. Until the humaneness of all persons is recognized and respected, the risk of those defined as less than human will persist. Therefore, the lives of individuals with Down syndrome will remain vulnerable and tentative unless their value is fully acknowledged as being intrinsic to their humanity. Hence, it is imperative that society affirms the absolute fullness of their humanity and the absolute worth and sanctity of their lives.

We have to ensure that persons with Down syndrome be offered a status that observes their rights and privileges as citizens in a democratic society and, in a real sense, preserves their human dignity.

PART 2
OPTIONS FOR AN
INDEPENDENT LIFE

Chapter 2
People with Down Syndrome: Quality of Life and Future

JUAN PERERA

In developed countries, the concept of quality of life applied to planning and evaluation of services for disabled people was first used and studied only ten years ago (Goode 1990; Schalock et al. 1989). In countries in the process of development, it is practically impossible to talk about quality of life when all too frequently their preoccupations are focused on day-to-day survival, on the struggle to have human rights recognized and on obtaining basic health care, education, personal safety, work and daily subsistence (Fabian 1991).

The term 'quality of life' has gradually been introduced into the world of people with Down Syndrome because of three capital elements:

1. the application of the principle of normalization and its consequence, which is inclusion;
2. the longer life expectancy of people with Down syndrome;
3. the advances in scientific knowledge about the identity of the extra chromosome 21 and the specific consequences deriving from its presence.

This chapter revises the definitions and contents of the term 'quality of life', analyses different models of research into this subject and details the challenges that the specific associations, professionals and parents face in order to improve the quality of life for people with Down syndrome on the threshold of the third millennium.

Definitions of Quality of Life

The term 'quality of life' is a common and undeniably topical expression that is used in the field of marketing, in political language, in colloquial speech and, of course, in the scientific field. The idea of quality of life is associated with different elements that have as a common denominator a positive significance: comfort, welfare, good standard of living, satisfaction, happiness (Casas 1993).

There is not a simple definition of the term, and researchers are agreed that any evaluation of quality of life is essentially subjective (Blatt 1987; Edgerton 1990; Schalock 1990; Taylor and Racino 1991). The following are among the definitions offered in the last decade (Dennis et al. 1993):

- satisfaction with one's luck in life and a sense of satisfaction with one's own experiences of the world (Taylor and Bogden 1990);
- a sense of satisfaction that is more than contentment or happiness (Coulter 1990);
- a general well being that is synonymous with a general satisfaction with life, happiness, contentment or success (Stark and Goldsbury 1990);
- the ability to adopt a lifestyle that fulfils one's own wishes and needs (Karen et al. 1990).

Blatt (1987) emphasizes the temporary, relative and individual nature of quality of life. Goode (1990) refers to various principles in relation to disabled people's quality of life and the providers of services identified the following principles:

1. The quality of life for people with disabilities is composed of the same factors and relations as those that appear to be important for people without a disability.
2. Quality of life is experienced when a person's basic needs have been satisfied and when they have the opportunity to propose and achieve goals in the principal areas of life.
3. The meaning of quality of life in the principal facets of life can be validated by consensual means with a wide group of people who represent the points of view of the disabled, their families, professionals, providers of services, lawyers and others.
4. An individual's quality of life is intrinsically related to other people's quality of life in his or her environment.
5. A person's quality of life reflects the cultural heritage of that person and of those who are around him or her.

Many researchers concur that the quality of life for people with a disability is comprised of the same elements as the quality of life for people without a disability (Blatt 1987; Devereux 1988; Turnbull and Brunk 1990).

Goode (1990) affirms that the concept of quality includes the same factors for everyone. Brown (1998) says that it can be analysed according to the different types of disability and the age of the individuals, but the essential principles are applicable to different ages and disabled groups. Schalock et al. (1989) also maintain that the construct of quality of life is essentially the same whether people have disabilities or not, and that everyone has the same capacities and wishes for affiliation, a sense of what is valuable and giving importance to taking decisions. Flanagan (1976), for his part, suggests that when we try to evaluate the dimensional structure involved in the concept of quality of life, we should make some adjustments to take into account the limits imposed by disabilities. Borthwick-Duffy (1992) maintains that in the case of people with mental retardation, comparisons of quality of life have to be made only within homogeneous groups of people, that is to say, taking variables such as age, level of cognitive development and state of health into consideration. In any event, it does appear that one should be careful when dealing with this subject in disabled people and not assume that they present exactly the same characteristics as other types of population (Dennis et al. 1993). However, Taylor and Racino (1991) are of the opinion that throughout time philosophers have failed in their attempt to reach agreement over the meaning of the concept of quality of life. They recommend being cautious, since describing such a complex subject within the field of disabled people is not so easy as for other populations. Because of the many different ways of focusing the approach to quality of life, it is necessary to resort to an extensive literature in order to understand and have the right perspective in relation to the quality of life for people with a disability.

Worthy of special attention is the concept 'optimum theory' discussed by Speight et al. (1991) and applied in the clinical and developmental literature. The optimum theory suggests a holistic point of view on health and well-being which provides a balance between the values of diversity and the values of universality. Speight et al. suggest that by adopting an optimum world point of view we can advance beyond the fragmented point of view of individuals who have different external realities and aims, and we thereby reach a more global point of view. Their model describes an individual's vision of the world as a Venn diagram represented by three circles: the individual, human universality and cultural specificity. They suggested that the neuralgic point was situated in the area of intersection between the three defined spheres, as it is only in their interaction that we can begin to understand the mixture of influences on individuals' points of view of the world.

It is clear from this review that quality of life is a pluridimensional concept which does, of course, include the behaviour of the individual in response to a number of *ecological domains* that affect him or her (Evans et al. 1985).

Schalock (1997) focuses the concept of quality of life on programmes for the disabled in the twenty-first century. With his characteristic brilliance and clarity, he stresses four important changes:

1. A new vision of what the options of life involve for people with a disability. This vision includes a special emphasis on the person's vigour and capacities, on the importance of a normalized environment,

on the application of appropriate services according to the person's age, on the development of individualized support systems, on greater adaptive functioning and the development of a role or social status and on the increase in confidence in the person's own possibilities (Luckasson et al. 1992).
2. Matching the concepts of quality of life with an increase and guarantees of quality, with improved control and with an evaluation based on the results (Albin 1992; Schalock 1994b, c).
3. Focusing efforts on the principal areas of vital activity and on the fact that a functional limitation only becomes a disability through interaction with the demands of the environment (Institute of Medicine 1991). Thus, the spotlight of (re)habilitation should be centred on reducing the functional limitations of people and therefore on reducing the associated disabilities.
4. A paradigm based on the supports usually reflected in work programmes and home support (Bradley et al. 1994) and in individualized planning, centred on the person.

Schalock (1997) was of the opinion that programmes for the disabled in the twenty-first century will be guided by four characteristics:

1. a change in the conception of the disability;
2. they will be centred on quality of life;
3. services will be based on the supports;
4. the critical importance of valued, person-referenced outcomes.

This perspective is especially important when the conception of the disability (in our case the mental retardation of the person with Down syndrome) has already evolved from a perspective centred on services towards one that is centred on persons.

The American Association of Mental Retardation proposed this definition of mental retardation (Luckasson et al. 1992):

> Mental retardation refers to substantial limitations in the actual functioning. It is characterized by an intellectual functioning significantly inferior to the average, which generally coexists together with limitations in two or more of the following areas of adaptation skills: communication, self-care, life in the home, social skills, utilization of the community, self-management, health and safety, functional academic abilities, free time and work. The mental retardation should manifest itself before 18 years. (p. 1)

This definition involves a change of paradigm that is directly linked to the concept of quality of life: instead of being limited to studying the individual and acting upon him or her, *it is also necessary to evaluate and act upon the environment in which that individual is integrated*.

From being considered as an absolute feature of the individual, the mental retardation becomes an expression of the interaction between the person with a limited intellectual functioning and his or her environment.

The essential task of professionals is not limited to making a diagnosis, classifying individuals with a mental retardation from a medical perspective and with this information determining the treatments and services required, *but* also includes evaluating them multidimensionally on the basis of their interaction with the contexts in which they move; and on the basis of that individual's evaluation and environment, determining his or her special educational needs. To do this, subjects will not be classified according to their IQ, but the type and intensity of the supports needed will be determined. In this way, instead of establishing a system of classification based on the subject's intelligence levels (slight, average, severe, profound), a reference system is proposed that is based on the intensity of the supports required by the persons with mental retardation (limited, intermittent, extensive, generalized).

Four different dimensions of evaluation are approached: a) intellectual functioning and adaptive skills; b) psychological-emotional considerations; c) physical, health and etiological considerations; and d) environmental considerations.

Bearing in mind these four dimensions, the process of *evaluation is structured* on a series of steps that begin with the differential valuation of the mental retardation, *continues* with the valuation and description of the subject based on the potentials and limitations in the different dimensions and in relation to the environment in which he or she moves; and *ends* with the determination of the necessary supports in each one of the proposed dimensions.

Schalock (1994a, b, c) also indicates four courses of action that are derived from the aforementioned characteristics in programmes for the disabled in the coming twenty-first century:

1. Begin with the end in mind:
   - establish programme models and funding streams that have a high probability of producing valued, person-referenced outcomes;
   - establish agreed quality of life areas such as: rights and dignity, individual control, community membership, relationships, personal growth, and accomplishment and well being.
2. Operationalize the supports model:
   - develop quantitative measures of support levels;
   - Develop support standards.
3. Restructure the service delivery system:
   - implement a service delivery system built upon a matrix of major life activity areas and support intensities;

- change the current system from a downstream, deficit model to an upstream, growth and development model;
- base funding mechanisms on the support needs of the person;
- measure valued, person-referenced outcomes.
3. Capitalize on the entrepreneurial spirit:
    - recognize the 'three Cs' of the twenty-first century: customer first, competition and change;
    - be entrepreneurs.

Quality of Life Research Models

The forms of theoretically focusing quality of life in the field of social research are very different (Bradley and Knoll 1990; Speight et al. 1991). The argument of the objective focus versus the subjective focus is one of the latest topics (Cummins 1997). Some researchers try to objectify and quantify quality of life (Stark and Goldsbury 1990), while others believe that quality of life is, because of its very nature, a unique, individual and subjective concept that resists objective measurement and demands qualitative approaches (Edgerton 1990). Many others use a combination of these approaches with the aim of increasing knowledge of the quality of life (Bradley and Knoll 1990; Cameto 1990; Conroy and Feinstein 1990; Schalock 1994a). Cummins (1993a, b, c) proposes in his comprehensive Quality of Life Scale that it has to be researched and measured separately.

Quantitative models

For more than 50 years social researchers have used *quantitative approaches* in research on the quality of life. However, their use in research on the quality of life for people with a disability is a more recent phenomenon (Stark and Goldsbury 1990). The principal objective of the quantification of quality of life for people with or without a disability has been to compare and plan services, programmes and policies referring to the quality of life for specific populations. The social researchers have studied quality of life indicators using different approaches:

- study of the social indicators;
- study of psychological indicators;
- ecological analysis.

Studies of *social indicators* generally measure the collective quality of life of groups or populations. They refer to external conditions, based on the environment, such as health, social welfare, friendship, living standards, home, public health, education, work, taxation, family, children (Cameto 1990; Roessler 1990). These indicators are frequently considered insufficient to evaluate individual quality of life or to evaluate the results of services because they only reflect the judgement of an independent person, prompted by external factors. These indicators do not consider individual psychological experiences of satisfaction that cannot be correlated to external conditions (Campbell et al. 1979).

Studies of *psychological indicators* research and measure the subjective reactions of the individual to the presence or absence of certain life experiences. They are centred on psychological well-being and personal satisfaction. Dimity (1997) believes that there are four basic psychological components in quality of life:

1. knowledge of or 'knowing' an individual;
2. an understanding of their circumstances;
3. some insight into how they experience their circumstances;
4. a reflection of such experiences against the current mores or values of the culture.

The social and psychological indicators of quality of life in disabled people have been studied in relation to residential programmes, working and social relations, employment with support, medical rehabilitation programmes and so on (Hasazi et al. 1992; Wehman et al. 1987).

Schalock (1994c) points out that social and psychological indicators have no correlation between themselves nor with a global evaluation of quality of life. He recommended the use of *ecological analysis* in order to measure the correctness of the adjustment between the environment and the subject's resources or stresses. From an ecological perspective, quality of life is optimum when the needs and wishes of the individual are attended to by society and the subject has the suitable resources to confront the demands of the environment (Cameto 1990). Other researchers have proposed that a quality of life index be used to measure the result of the services, and as a criterion of the right adaptation between individuals and their environments (Murrell and Norris 1983). Along these lines Brown et al. (1989) contribute the idea that quality of life is the interaction between the individual and his or her environment, which can be described in terms of the individual's personal control over the environment.

Methodology in quality of life quantitative research

Quantitative methodologies to evaluate quality of life use objective and subjective measures, self-reports and questionnaires to other family members, as well as interviews and surveys. Some researchers use a combination of methods. The self-reports have the advantage of collecting direct quality of life factors that are important for the person concerned. However, this is problematical, for example, in people with Down syndrome because owing to their mental retardation they lack a set of experiences with which to compose their own quality of life experiences.

Also, they have difficulties in forming judgements and communicating their points of view. These problems have led some researchers to adapt the instruments of evaluation by simplifying the choice of answers (Heal and Sigelman 1990; Newton et al. 1991).

The use of questionnaires for family members, caregivers or friends solves some of the problems of the self-reports, but other people's perceptions are not necessarily the same as the ones that the subjects have of their own quality of life.

It would seem reasonable to propose, therefore, that through the use of a combination of methods (for example, self-reports, questionnaires from family members, participatory research) the quantitative methodologies could begin to solve problems related to the definition of quality of life, the potential bias on the part of researchers and the quality of life of subjects in relation to that of other groups surrounding them. Nevertheless, it is not quite so clear that quantitative methodologies can be constructed to provide a more adequate solution to the problem of quality of life factors being temporary and influenced by the context.

Qualitative models

The qualitative approach in research on quality of life assumes that by listening to disabled persons talk about their experiences, we can better understand the problems they face and we can design services to support them more efficiently (Bogden and Taylor 1982; Covert and Carr 1988; Crutcher 1990; Devereux 1988). Edgerton (1990) affirmed that any discussion on quality of life is culturally and individually interpreted by both the researcher and the one who responds, and he is inclined towards ethnographic, naturalist and longitudinal studies of quality of life. The qualitative approach would appear to have the advantages of considering a subject's quality of life in relation to that of those around him, as well as its temporary and contextual nature. The qualitative descriptions of disabled people's quality of life are, however, generally limited by definition.

The controversy between qualitative and quantitative researchers begins to be overcome when Goode (1994) affirms that any evaluation of an individual's quality of life must contain objective and subjective elements and that there can be differences between them. Also, that it should have a relational or social component which is neither 'objective' nor 'subjective', but which reflects the fact that the individual is immersed in social relations. In short, the difference between the objective and subjective data is a question of degree and not of quality.

The revision of present methodologies, both qualitative as well as quantitative, being used in quality of life research suggests that a relation of cooperation should be established in its level of application (Goode 1997).

Cummins (1997) references more than one hundred scales being used today to measure quality of life. Some of these instruments are based on structures that clearly specify a concept of quality of life and are developed on sophisticated psychometric systems. They frequently measure both subjective and objective components of quality of life. The elements most frequently evaluated in the quality of life scales are: life in the home and in the community; economy (employment/properties); social integration (family, friends, supports); state of health/safety; personal control and capacity to decide (Schalock 1994b).

A Comprehensive Definition of Quality of Life

On reaching this point it would seem necessary to establish with Cummins (1997) a comprehensive definition of quality of life: 'Quality of life is both objective and subjective, each axis being the aggregate of seven domains: material well-being, productivity, intimacy, safety, community and emotional well-being. Subjective domains comprise satisfaction weighted by their importance to the individual.'

The reader interested in this subject should consult the *Directory of Instruments to Measure Quality of Life and Cognate Areas* (Cummins 1995). Because of its interest and application to the world of the disabled, in the widest sense of the term, the scales that deserve emphasizing are those of Bellamy et al. (1990), Bigelow et al. (1991), Cummins (1993a, b, c), Lehman (1988), Schalock and Keith (1993), Skantze et al. (1992).

Quality of Life and Down Syndrome

To talk about quality of life would not have made much sense 50 years ago when the life expectancy for people with Down syndrome did not exceed 23 years. Nowadays in developed countries the majority of people with Down syndrome (Steele 1996) are young people or adults who have looked after their health, have benefited from early attention programmes, have attended inclusive school and have faced adult life with the same desires and aspirations as any young person of their age. That is why it makes a lot of sense to talk about quality of life with a fundamental objective: to *achieve maximum personal autonomy*.

Today we are faced with the challenge of adult life. As soon as basic health needs have been covered, it is necessary for society to develop educational and social services that are gradually addressed towards adult life, so that an interaction is produced whereby a reform takes place in the services that can improve quality of life (Perera 1997).

It is important therefore to be aware that effective quality of life programmes for people with Down syndrome have to have a *perspective that covers the whole of the individual's life* and especially as an adult. *This cannot be improvised.* One cannot demand an adult to do what they have not had the chance of doing as a child or young person; what is acquired during the first stages of life determines, to a certain extent, what is going to happen later. If a child has been overprotected during the first years of life and has not had the advantages of a wide range of stimulation, that child in adult life will reach lower levels of adaptation and autonomy. For this reason the best preparation for adult life is providing effective and quality services during the early years of life. Our inclusive schools still leave much to be desired. In many cases they lack the necessary supports and a systematic stimulation of language that allows friendships to develop in the community in which they live, all of which are tools for adult life (Perera and Rondal 1995).

It is important for families to be aware that inclusion is not only a problem of being included in schools, but it is also a problem of being included at home and in the community in which they live. The family has to be a platform of integration and not a nucleus of overprotection (Perera 1993). To note a few examples: Timmons and Brown (1996) have found how young disabled people are told to go to bed earlier than those who are not disabled. It has also been shown that they have fewer friends, they do not go out to eat with other children so often and they receive money only if they ask for it and without any rules or duties in return. The result is that young people stagnate *because we try to give them solutions and comfort rather than giving them exploration and stimulation opportunities*. These explorations play an important role in the biological development of the brain and, consequently, on the social and cognitive configuration of their adult status.

There are today extremely important works that promote adult life. Denholm (1992) writes that young disabled people have the same aspirations for friends, relationships, fashion, moral codes and so on as young people without any disability. Their aspirations are the same, but they have fewer opportunities to achieve these aspirations. *This has to change*.

Many authors show that the disabled, and people with Down syndrome in particular, tend to enjoy a shorter and less varied leisure time. Brown et al. (1992) show that this becomes more noticeable in people with Down syndrome after they reach 25. Reid and Block (1996) are of the opinion that opportunities for leisure, the autonomy of displacement and physical care form part of the adult's social schemes. Women with Down syndrome seem to achieve greater effectiveness than men in a wide range of activities, although it would also appear that they are more protected than men.

One thing is clear: with better opportunities to express their wishes and likings and with the ability to take decisions in a normalized environment, people with Down syndrome are more prepared for adult life. *The opportunity to choose is a basic criterion in quality of life models* (Brown 1997).

Up to here I have emphasized some attitudes that are important for the development of young people with Down syndrome when they approach adulthood. I have included them in a quality of life model and I have emphasized the need for a holistic consideration, the approach to the total life-cycle, the development of the capacity to choose and the need to develop a positive self-image.

But there is more. In this chapter I would like to draw attention to the need for associations, parents and professionals to work together in drawing up quality of life programmes by the hand of experts. As we have seen above, we have well-defined dimensions, indicators and methods of research into quality of life. We have analysed the important change that has taken place in the definition of mental retardation. Now what is needed is for us to be capable of changing our attitude and for things to be clear to those of us who have - to a certain extent - the responsibility of seeing into the future and producing solutions.

The Key Points for People with Down Syndrome at the Start of the Twenty-first Century

As an organized world movement representative of those with Down syndrome we have an obligation to promote before the international organizations (the UN, UNESCO, WHO and so on) recognition of the rights of adult life with a strong emphasis on the principle of non-discrimination.

Health

This begins with the right to health. It is vitally important that a person with Down syndrome - the same as any other person - enjoys the best health possible. We are today in a position to be able to predict, in most cases, what disturbances may appear and at what time in life. That is why the application of preventive medicine programmes by means of regular and systematic examinations is so important, because through them we can prevent and correct any health problems as soon as they appear.

But we have to pay attention to the criteria of distributing health resources in different countries. One of the three bioethical principles as regards health resources is that of justice, which is usually formulated in the following manner: 'The same cases demand the same treatments' (Gafo 1994, p. 10). It is unjust to discriminate against a person for reasons of sex, race, religion, financial position, disability and so on.

This has special significance in the case of organ transplants. The criterion for distributing this health resource cannot be either merit or prestige or financial position; 'the same cases demand the same treatments'. A Nobel prize winner, football player or a person with Down syndrome has the same right to a transplant.

However, there are authors who consider that the criterion 'the same cases demand the same treatments' should be complemented with that of preferential treatment to the poorest and weakest (Amor 1995), as society inevitably tends to give less attention to its most financially needy, most culturally neglected and most socially deprived groups.

A society's maturity and development is measured, among other variables, by the attention given to its most financially, socially or culturally underprivileged. To have a supernumerary chromosome and consequently a mental retardation means having a limitation. But because a person's worth in life is not measured by the intelligence quotient, it is unjust to deny a transplant to a person with Down syndrome when that person needs it.

Social image

This is another important point which needs action: the need to improve the social image of people with Down syndrome. Expressions such as 'people who suffer from', are 'afflicted with' or are 'victims of' Down syndrome should disappear from our lexicon. We should stop unconsciously seeing the person with Down syndrome as someone who is sick. We should stop talking about illness. Claudia Werneck (1997) affirms: 'in popular fantasy, illness gives the idea of contagion, it suggests that people with Down syndrome are not healthy because they are ill' (p. 17). And this is absolutely false. Down syndrome is a unique form of being and living in the world, which is determined genetically and from which we so-called 'normal' people have a lot to learn (Perera 1996).

The social image of a person is the culture medium that creates quality of life. We psychologists know that the recognition and esteem of those around us produces personal satisfaction and equilibrium. Rejection, on the other hand, produces anxiety and depression. It is necessary to change social attitudes and proclaim a plural and modern society, enriched with diversity.

Self-advocacy

Another important aspect and one that is often neglected in many places of the world is what is called self-advocacy. The People First organization in the United Kingdom announced that the conclusions of a recent congress staged by and for people with Down syndrome were as follows:

> The right to life; that they themselves should know about Down syndrome and teach others about it, not to be treated as children, the right to respect towards their lives and their persons; to speak for themselves, to be a part of our community in conditions of equality, to do what they want to do and not what others say that they have to do; to take decisions; to have and to enjoy their own feelings and opinions; not to be intimidated, hurt or badly treated, to have sexual relations if they want; to have a child and to keep it; to have a proper job and salary; to be independent with the necessary support; to have their own friends and social life; to have access to information making it easy to understand; to learn from their own mistakes; to assume responsibilities. (unpublished document)

This declaration should give us cause for reflection. We are on the wrong path if we tell people with Down syndrome what they have to do and then ask if they have done it well. We should listen to them more, include them as active members on the committees of our associations and help them to explain their feelings and opinions.

Work

Parents and professionals also need to consider the importance of work in the adult life of the person with Down syndrome as a source of equilibrium and quality of life. Quality of life also means having a plan for the future (Perera 1993), and one cannot have a plan for the future without a stable paid job. The majority of people with Down syndrome are today capable of work if they are properly trained, if we adapt jobs to their real needs and if we give them the opportunity to do them. Experiences in this field show that work transforms their lives, enriches their personal experiences and gives them greater security and autonomy. At present it is possible that most of them will outlive their parents and that their brothers and sisters cannot, or do not want to, look after them. This has to be anticipated and prepared for from childhood. They have to be trained for work. The person who is working has more probabilities of being self-sufficient, of living independently or in supervised homes without being a burden to the family and to society.

Partnership and marriage

Lastly, two important aspects of adult life that are gaining strength in the movement for Down syndrome: partnership and marriage.

Brown (1996) analyses the advantages of living with a partner for people with Down syndrome. First, they have a friend and companion with whom they can share a vast range of experiences and social learning, which generates a positive adaptation. Language and interests are also stimulated. Very important too is the affective complement that they mutually impart to one another. This balances the personality of both, gives them autonomy and strength to overcome difficulties and in some cases has the natural result of sexual surrender and satisfaction.

The greater the disability, the greater the need for help and support. Partnership fills this need for help and support and, in short, for companionship. When speaking to young people and adults with Down syndrome their desires to get married are clearly perceived. Why should someone with Down syndrome be condemned to live alone when this is not what they want?

People with Down syndrome generally seek companions with some disability. Being aware that those companions have limitations, they feel more comfortable. In most cases, because of their opinions or beliefs, it is the parents and professionals who do not allow a relationship to develop between people with Down syndrome.

It is obvious that parents and professionals have to be concerned about training them in everything connected with affectivity and sexuality. There are good training programmes on this subject and it is necessary to apply them carefully when the time comes. It is also important that partnership is complemented with sharing the work in the home and with a good training in domestic tasks. A certain amount of supervision has to be planned, which can be withdrawn as and when the couple mature.

Among partners with Down syndrome who live together there is frequently a degree of mutual understanding between them which is based on affection and support. Some receive external support from specialized staff. Others live in apartments attached to the houses of their families. Even those partners who have separated say that they have become stronger after the marital experience.

One thing is clear: if we admit the fact that people with Down syndrome are taking on the roles of adults, we have to recognize that one of these roles is in partnership or in marriage.

Conclusion

The reality is that today the good quality-of-life programmes for people with Down syndrome are creating a situation in which they enjoy good health and a longer life, that they have social recognition, are educated in an ordinary school, are trained for work, live integrated in the community, are capable of self-advocacy and, in short, have their own plans for the future. In countries in the process of development, where there is still much to be done, it is important that they have a clear model to follow, objectives to achieve and unconditional support from the more advanced societies.

However, although 'When dreams come true' was the slogan for the recent VI World Congress on Down Syndrome in Madrid, whose papers have been the basis for this book, not all dreams do come true or, perhaps, there are other realities one must try to reach.

Today people with Down syndrome who have a decent job, who are truly autonomous or who are living with a partner are a minority. Furthermore, dreams are sometimes unattainable goals. Not attaining them does not mean failing. There are some young people who, because they have limitations or medical problems associated with Down syndrome will never reach the ideal standard, but who in their own way and with their limited capacities developed to the full, will also make dreams come true (true in a different way). These dreams have to be discussed too, and above all it must be explained to the families. What matters is the endeavour. To be clear about the model to follow and the objectives to be reached ... even though they may never be.

References

Albin JM (1992). Quality Improvement in Employment and Other Human Services: Managing for Quality though Change. Baltimore MD: Brookes.

Amor JR (1995) Ética y Deficiencia Mental. Madrid: Universidad Pontificia de Comillas.

Bellamy GT, Newton JS, Lebaron NM, Homer RH (1990) Quality of life and life style outcomes: a challenge for residential programmes. In Schalock RL (ed) Quality of Life: Perspectives and Issues. Washington DC: American Association on Mental Retardation.

Bigelow DA, Gareau MJ, Young DI (1991) Quality of Life Questionnaire. (a) Interviewer rating version (b) Respondent self-report version. Oregon: Western Mental Health Research Center.

Blatt B (1987). The Conquest of Mental Retardation. Austin, TX: Pro-Ed.

Bogden R, Taylor S (1982) Inside Out: The Social Meaning of Mental Retardation. Toronto: University of Toronto Press.

Borthwick-Duffy SA (1992) Quality of life and quality of care in mental retardation. In Rowitz L (ed) Mental Retardation in the Year 2000. New York: Springer-Verlag. pp. 52-66.

Bradley VJ, Ashbaugh JW, Blaney BC (1994) Creating Individual Supports for People with Developmental Disabilities: A Mandate for Change at Many Levels. Baltimore MD: Brookes.

Bradley VJ, Knoll J (1990) Shifting Paradigm in Services to People with Developmental Disabilities. Cambridge, MA: Human Research Institute.

Brown RI (1996) Partnership and Marriage in Down Syndrome. Conference in Rome at the International Conference on Down Syndrome, organized by Associazione Italiana Persone Down.

Brown RI (1997) Quality of Life for People with Disabilities: Models, Research and Practice. Cheltenham: Stanley Thornes.

Brown RI (1998) Quality of Life for Handicapped People. London: Croom Helm.

Brown RI, Bayer I, Brown R (1992) Empowerment and Development Handicaps: Choices and Quality of Life. Toronto: Captus Press; London: Chapman and Hall.

Brown RI, Bayer MB, MacFarlane C (1989) Rehabilitation Programmes: Performance and Quality of Life of Adults with Developmental Handicaps. Toronto: Lugus.

Cameto R (1990) Quality of Life: its Conceptualization and Use as a Tool for Social Policy. Unpublished manuscript, San Francisco State University and the University of California, Berkeley.

Campbell A, Converse PE, Rodgers WL (1979) The Quality of American Life. New York: Sage.

Casas F (1993) El concepto de calidad de vida en la intervención social en el ámbito de la infancia. In Proceedings of the III Jornadas de Psicología de la Intervención Social, vol. 2. Madrid: Ministerio de Asuntos Sociales, Inserso. pp. 649-72.

Conroy J, Feinstein C (1990) Measuring quality of life: where have we been, where are we going?. In Schalock RL, Bogale MJ (eds) Quality of Life: Perspectives and Issues. Washington DC: American Association on Mental Retardation. pp. 227-34.

Coulter D (1990) Home is the place: quality of life for young children with developmental disabilities. In Schalock RL, Bogale MJ (eds) Quality of Life: Perspectives and Issues. Washington DC: American Association on Mental Retardation. pp. 61-70.

Covert A, Carr T (eds) (1988) Valued Based Services for Young Adults with Deaf-blindness. Sands Point, NY: Hellen Keller National Center for Deaf Blind Youths and Adults Technical Assistance Center in cooperation with the Association for Persons with Severe Handicaps.

Crutcher D (1990) Quality of life versus quality of life judgements: a parent's perspective. In Schalock RL, Bogale MJ (eds) Quality of Life: Perspectives and Issues. Washington DC: American Association on Mental Retardation. pp. 17-22.

Cummins RA (1993a) The Comprehensive Quality of Life Scale - Adult, 4th edn. Melbourne: School of Psychology, Deakin University.

Cummins RA (1993b) The Comprehensive Quality of Life Scale - Adolescents, 4th edn. Melbourne: School of Psychology, Deakin University.

Cummins, RA (1993c) The Comprehensive Quality of Life Scale - Intellectual Disability, 4th edn. Melbourne: School of Psychology, Deakin University.

Cummins RA (1995) Directory of Instruments to Measure Quality of Life and Cognate Areas. Melbourne: School of Psychology, Deakin University.

Cummins RA (1997) Assessing quality of life. In Brown RI (ed) Quality of Life for People with Disabilities. Cheltenham: Stanley Thornes.

Denholm C (1992) Developmental Needs of Adolescents: Application to Adolescents with Down Syndrome. The National Conference of the Canadian Down Syndrome Society. Calgary: Canadian Down Syndrome Society, University of Calgary.

Dennis R, Williams W, Giangreco M, Cloninger C (1993) Calidad de vida como contexto de planificación y evaluación de servicios para personas con discapacidad. Exceptional Children 59, 6: 499-512.

Devereux A (1988) Valued based services: a parent perspective. In Covert A, Carr T (eds) Value Based Services for Young Adults with Deaf-Blindness. Sands Point, NY: Hellen Keller National Center for Deaf Blind Youths and Adults Technical Assistance Center, in cooperation with the Association for Persons with Severe Handicaps. pp. 23-6.

Dimity P (1997) A focus on the individual, theory and reality: making the connection through the lives of individuals. In Brown RI (ed) Quality of Life for People with Disabilities. Cheltenham: Stanley Thornes.

Edgerton R (1990) Quality of life from a longitudinal research perspective. In Schalock RL, Bogale MJ (eds) Quality of Life: Perspectives and Issues. Washington DC: American Association on Mental Retardation. pp. 149-60.

Evans DR, Burns JE, Robinson WE, Garret OJ (1985) The quality of life questionnaire: a multidimensional measure. American Journal of Community Psychology 13: 305-22.

Fabian E (1991) Using quality of life indicators in rehabilitation program evaluation. Rehabilitation Counseling Bulletin 34, 4: 334-56.

Flanagan P (1976) A research approach to improving our quality of life. American Psychologist 33: 305-22.

Gafo J (1994) Aspectos Biomédicos e Implicaciones Éticas. Madrid: Universidad Pontificia de Comillas.

Goode D (1990) Thinking about and discussing quality of life. In Schalock RL, Bogale MJ (eds) Quality of Life: Perspectives and Issues. Washington, DC: American Association on Mental Retardation. pp. 41-58.

Goode DA (ed) (1994) Quality of Life for Persons with Disabilities: International Perspectives and Issues. Cambridge, MA: Brooklin Books.

Goode DA (1997) Assessing the quality of life of adults with profound disabilities. In Brown RI (ed) Quality of Life for People with Disabilities. Cheltenham: Stanley Thornes.

Hasazi S, Hock M, Gravedi-Cheng L (1992) Vermont's post-school indicators: utilizing satisfaction and post-school outcomes data for program improvement. In Rusch F, DeStefano L (eds) Transition from School to Work for Youth and Adults with Disability. Sycamore, IL: Sycamore. pp. 485-506.

Heal L, Sigelman C (1990) Methodological issues in measuring quality of life of individuals with mental retardation. In Schalock, RL, Bogale, MJ (eds) Quality of Life: Perspectives and Issues. Washington DC: American Association on Mental Retardation. pp. 161-76).

Institute of Medicine (1991) Disability in America: Toward a National Agenda for Prevention. Washington DC: Academy Press.

Karen O, Lambour G, Greespan S (1990) Persons in transition. In Schalock RL, Bogale MJ (eds) Quality of Life: Perspectives and Issues. Washington DC: American Association on Mental Retardation. pp. 95-92.

Lehman AF (1988) A quality of life interview for the chronically mentally ill. Evaluation and Program Planning 11: 51-62.

Luckasson R, Coulter DL, Polloway EA, Reiss S, Schalock RI, Snell MI, Spitalnik DM, Stark JA (1992) Mental Retardation: Definition, Classification and Systems of Supports. Washington DC: American Association on Mental Retardation.

Murrel SA, Norris FH (1983) Quality of life as the criterion for need assessment and community psychology. Journal of Community Psychology 11: 88-97.

Newton JS, Horner RH, Lund L (1991) Honoring activity preferences in individualized plan development: A descriptive analysis. Journal of the Association for Persons with Severe Disabilities 16, 4: 207-12.

Perera J (1993) Síndrome de Down. Programa de Acción Educativa. Madrid: Ciencias de la Educación Preescolar y Especial (CEPE).

Perera J (1996) Calidad de vida para las personas con Síndrome de Down: ¿qué significa?. Revista Down 6: 30.

Perera J (1997) Social and Labour Integration for People with Down's Syndrome. In Rondal JA, Perera J, Nadel,L, Comblain A (eds) Down's Syndrome: Psychological, Psychobiological and Socio-educational Perspectives. London: Whurr. pp. 219-33.

Perera J, Rondal JA (1995) Cómo hacer hablar al niño con Síndrome de Down y mejorar su lenguaje. Un programa de intervención psicolingüística. Madrid: Ciencias de la Educación Preescolar y Especial (CEPE).

Reid G, Block ME (1996) Motor development and physical education. In Stratford B, Gunn P (eds) New Approaches to Down Syndrome. London: Lussell.

Roessler R (1990) A quality of life perspective on rehabilitation counseling. Rehabilitation Counseling Bulletin 13, 2: 95-107.

Schalock, RL (1990) Where do we go from here? In Schalock RL, Bogale MJ (eds) Quality of Life: Perspectives and Issues. Washington DC: American Association on Mental Retardation. pp. 27-40.

Schalock RL (1994a) The concept of quality of life and its current applications in the field of mental retardation and development disabilities. In Goode D (ed) Quality of Life for Persons with Disabilities: International Perspectives and Issues. Cambridge MA: Brooklin Books.

Schalock RL (1994b) Promoting quality through quality enhancement techniques and outcome based evaluation. Journal on Developmental Disabilities 3: 1-16.

Schalock RL (1994c) Quality of life, quality enhancement and quality assurance: implications for programme planning and evaluation in the field of mental retardation and developmental disabilities. Evaluation and Programme Planning 17: 121-31.

Schalock RL (1997) The concept of quality of life in 21st century disability programmes. In Brown RI (ed) Quality of Life for People with Disabilities. Cheltenham: Stanley Thornes. pp. 327-40.

Schalock RL, Keith KD (1993) Quality of Life Questionnaire. Ohio: IDS Publishing Corporation.

Schalock RL, Keith KD, Hoffman K, Karen OC (1989) Quality of life, its measurement and us in human service programs. Mental Retardation 27, 1: 25-31.

Skantze K, Malm U, Dencker SJ, May PRA, Corrigan P (1992) Comparison of quality of life with standards of living in schizophrenic outpatients. British Journal of Psychiatry 161: 797-801.

Speight S, Myers L, Cox C, Highlen P (1991) A redefinition of multicultural counseling. Journal of Counseling and Development 70: 29-36.

Stark J, Goldsbury T (1990) Quality of life from childhood to adulthood. In Schalock RL, Bogale MJ (eds) Quality of Life: Perspectives and Issues. Washington DC: American Association on Mental Retardation. pp. 71-84.

Steele J (1996) Epidemiology: incidence, prevalence and size of the Down Syndrome population. In Stratford B, Gunn P (eds) New Approaches to Down Syndrome. London: Lussell.

Taylor S, Bogden R (1990) Quality of life and the individual's perspective. In Schalock RL, Bogale MJ (eds) Quality of Life: Perspectives and Issues. Washington, DC: American Association on Mental Retardation. pp. 27-40.

Taylor S, Racino A (1991) Community living: lessons for today. In Meyer E, Peck C, Brown L (eds) Critical Issues in the Lives of People with Severe Disabilities. Baltimore MD: Brookes. pp. 235-8.

Timmons V, Brown RI (1996) Quality of life - issues for children with handicaps. In Brown RI (ed) Quality of Life for People with Disabilities: Models, Research and Practice. London: Chapman & Hall.

Turnbull HR, Brunk G (1990) Quality of life and public philosophy. In Schalock RL, Bogale MJ (eds) Quality of Life: Perspectives and Issues. Washington, DC: American Association on Mental Retardation. pp. 193-210.

Wehman P, Moon S, Everson J, Wood W, Barcus, J (1987) Transition from School to Work. New Challenges for Youth with Severe Disabilities. Baltimore MD: Brookes.

Werneck C (1997) Nosotros somos la próxima noticia. Conferencia pronunciada en el VI Congreso Mundial sobre el Síndrome de Down. Madrid: Fundación ONCE (en prensa).

Chapter 3
A Working Role and Full Citizenship for the Adult with Down Syndrome

ENRICO MONTOBBIO

I believe I have been asked to write this chapter because I am in charge of running a research centre that has, in the last few years, found work placement for around 600 young people with learning disabilities in the open labour market in the city of Genova, Italy.

Among this group around 10 per cent are part of what I call the great and heterogeneous family of Dr Down. Each of these young men and women has been 'accompanied' individually in the workplace and followed indirectly for many months. My observations and experience have left a deep mark, and meaningfully modified my 'world map'. I have learned more from this experience than I can teach in turn.

I would like to acknowledge, by way of introduction, my thankfulness to the young people I have worked with and their parents, who have been 'chosen by lot' (as Kundera would say) by God's computer. They experience directly this particular human condition that is being somebody with Down syndrome, or having a child with Down syndrome.

I think it is also important to state at the outset that the inclusion of people with learning disabilities in normal, open work placements is standard practice in many regional districts in Italy. Recently, a national research project organized by our Centro Studi (research centre) has allowed us to make a census of around 25,000 work placements that have been started in the last few years.

This article focuses on three main points:

1. the method used to allow inclusion into work of young people with Down syndrome and of other people with learning difficulties;
2. the justifications that lay behind the choices in methodology;
3. the results that have been achieved and what we have come to understand through our work.

The Methodology of Inclusion into Work

As a premise I would like to note that there are no substantial differences either in the method or in the characteristics of the 'learning to work' between young people with Down syndrome and other people with learning difficulties.

A colleague from Argentina (A Bauleo) has acutely observed that 'when there is an intention of planning the social inclusion of people with a difficulty, or of implementing different social models for the individual development (in this case of people with Down syndrome) it is necessary to include organizations for the mediation ... otherwise what is affirmed in the speeches about changing social structures will remain an ideological statement, showing good will but with no real impact' (personal communication). Implementing mediation has been our main achievement in Genova.

The world of learning disabilities is distant from the world of work, so much so that the two worlds usually don't meet spontaneously. Thus, in agreement with employers and unions, we decided to set up an 'area of mediation' that would make the subjectivity of people with disabilities compatible with the objectivity of the world of work (requirements, rules, company style and so on).

The main issue is bridging this gap - which can be very wide - so that a person with low skills who is unused to coping with standards becomes gradually (it's important to underline gradually) compatible with a system which usually requires high skills and high levels of standardization.

The area of mediation can be defined as a linking methodology that is placed between people with special needs and the world of work. The methodology must include professionals who are able to run projects for inclusion into work, instruments for the mediation process, and the possibility to form a team for the management of that process.

The availability of professionals and instruments for mediation was a specific request of employers before they agreed to collaborate in projects for the inclusion into work of young people with learning disabilities.

The professionals

The professionals are, in my opinion, the main element in the whole operation of inclusion of people with disabilities into the world of work. Their central position and the complexity of mediation require specific training and specific capacities. While we cannot go into a detailed analysis here, the elements that constitute such an interesting profession are the following:

* having specific competencies;
* operating full time on mediation;

- being able to work through projects after a precise commitment has been taken at the political level;
- being clearly recognized by public institutions and by the community.

Their tasks in dealing with the world of work include:

- researching possible jobs;
- researching support from employers;
- ergonomic analysis of tasks;
- supplying training to the group of workers in contact with the disabled worker;
- starting and monitoring the individual projects;
- managing chronic problems;

These tasks imply knowledge of work organization, and skills in negotiating, marketing and the ergonomic analysis of roles compatible with disability.

The tasks of the mediation professionals concerning the disabled people include:

- gathering requests;
- starting projects;
- assessing and evaluating young people with Down syndrome;
- planning intervention;
- choosing instruments of mediation;
- managing their inclusion in the work place.

These tasks require knowledge of the psychology of handicap, communication techniques, the capacity to handle relations with the disabled and their families, as well as the capacity to decide on assessment and on what instruments to use for mediation. Another important ability is the capacity to withstand the psychological stress of uncertainty and the possibility of failure.

In addition there are also a number of other tasks concerning what we call the secondary level of intervention. These refer to the necessary collaboration with public offices, government agencies, agencies and boards of education and training. Managing the entirety of these tasks requires the ability to work as part of a team, to network, and to accept responsibility.

The instruments for mediation

Insofar as the projects that must be used to complete the 'path' between school and work for young people with Down syndrome and other people with learning disabilities are concerned, I'd like to emphasize the necessity for organizations which aim to have good results in terms of quantity and quality to have at least three kinds of projects with different (although connected) objectives.

All projects are run within the normal world of work. The first is for younger people and in Italy is known as 'Tirocinio di Formazione in Situazione' (Apprenticeship for Training in the Setting). This training project involves a series of periods in different workplaces where the person can gain individual experience in the open world of work. Its general aim is to lead to greater maturity in all aspects of young people with Down syndrome, socialization through roles, and a gradual learning of working skills.

The second project, based in Genova, is called 'Borsa di Lavoro' (Work Grant) and is an instrument for mediation aimed at the employment of people with disabilities in the world of work. The young person with a disability is a 'guest' in the workplace for a year, during which he/she tries the job that he/she is going to take. This leads to a contract of employment at the end of the year. This is the most complex of the projects and requires that the young person with Down syndrome is able to:

- reach a sufficient maturity in relating to other people;
- acquire a good level of autonomy and appropriate socialization in the workplace;
- gain adequate working skills.

The third project, 'Inserimento Lavorativo Socio-Assistenziale' (Inclusion into Work for Socialization and Assistance), is dedicated to people with a more severe level of disability. This project makes it possible for people with severe disabilities to have permanent experience in open workplaces when their condition offers no possibility of employment. The aim is to offer a work opportunity even to people with Down syndrome who aren't able to reach a sufficient level of productivity, but who don't need a protected environment; it allows even those with great difficulties to have an active social role and a more acceptable identity. The candidates for this project are usually entitled to social benefits (which they don't lose), and the placements are set in the non-profit and public sectors.

I wish to emphasize, in ending this first section, that these projects have proved not only to be very effective, but also to be much less expensive in comparison with passive assistance in day centres or sheltered workshops.

The Reasons for the Choices of Method

Before exposing the results of the experience in Genova and the cultural reflections connected to our project I would like to make a few general, non-specialist remarks that constitute the background for the concept of our method.

First, the adult condition is established during childhood. For a good voyage through existence it is essential that one gets off to a good start.

Second, access to the adult world is made possible, at first, in the collective imagination. It is only if the community believes this access to be possible that a coherent life project and an effective curriculum for education and training can be implemented.

Third, a working role for young people with Down syndrome cannot ignore individual history and start at a predetermined age. Events that have taken place in earlier years deeply affect the emotional, educational and experiential growth of everyone. The facts I'm referring to here are only the 'normal' things that happen to all children; but they happen only with difficulty in the experience of people with Down syndrome.

Finally, I would like to point to the importance of the time factor. Changes, especially in the field of emotion and affection, are possible but very slow (for all men and women). It's not too difficult to teach a job to somebody with Down syndrome, but teaching them to work is very difficult. The former involves learning a sequence of operations (this can happen in a sheltered workshop), the latter involves acquiring a mentality, an attitude and the capacity for socialization at work, and also, of course, technical and practical skills. In addition, the latter requires time and a direct and prolonged experience of training in open work settings. The ability to work cannot be taught in an educational setting, but must be learnt in a workplace.

Results and Understandings

The results of the experience concerning the inclusion into work in the city of Genova are very positive both for people with learning disabilities in general and for the smaller group of people with Down syndrome .

The percentage of failure in the inclusion project is around 9 per cent, and it should be emphasized that this is never connected to cognitive problems (it's not that there are difficulties in learning a specific practical task), but rather with occasionally immature behaviour, which is not tolerated in the world of work (nor, generally speaking, in the adult world).

I consider it important to reflect on the fact that actions and speeches typically dedicated to people with Down syndrome are always centred on the mental representations interlocutors have of them. This is important at every age, but especially in the adult world, as each individual experiences the 'self' indirectly through the self-image one 'feels', 'perceives' and 'breathes' in other people with whom one interacts. This image, at first in 'micro' then in 'macro', supplies the structure for identity and the defensive mechanisms related to it.

It is self-evident that a young person with Down syndrome attending a specialized day centre will develop a self-image of 'handicapped person' and will behave as such, in an endlessly circular way. Through apprenticeship, and even more clearly through employment, young people with Down syndrome will be thought of as workers and will develop this image of themselves. The image of handicap will be gradually put aside, leading to a more positive identity. Such an identity will be based on these positive events and will bring young people as much as possible towards a more adult style of relationship.

Providing a role and the right to citizenship is the objective of our work. Both form the road that must gradually be followed to reach an adult identity. A young person with Down syndrome can take a working role only through a 'path of roles', a series of different experiences that become wider and more articulate, and are based on a continuous feedback between one's actions and other people's reactions. This means providing the opportunity for such young people to go through experiences and relations similar to those of other young men and women. It is important to recognize how rehabilitation usually makes it more difficult to experience realistic situations and the resulting relations, and therefore constitutes a psychological danger, especially if normal patterns are constantly denied for a long period of time. Rehabilitation, in fact, can even become a 'status', by which the person is seen as someone who is being constantly 'repaired'.

I would like to end by emphasizing again the results that are obtained by providing people with a working role. This role is a fundamental factor in personal identity; it is the main source for learning in the adult world (even the attention you are paying in reading these lines couldn't exist without the role you are playing); it is the main road to real socialization. The person who has no role is practically left out of society.

In the following quotation from Samuel Beckett can be found a message of faith in the possibilities of young people with Down syndrome:

> Where would I go if I could go,
> Who would I be if I could be,
> What would I say if I had a voice ...

Further Reading

Lepri C, Montobbio E (1993) Lavoro e Fasce Deboli. Milano: Franco Angeli.

Montobbio E (1992) Il Falso sè nell'Handicap Mentale. Pisa: Del Cerro.

Montobbio E (1994) Il Viaggio del Signor Down nel Mondo dei Grandi. Pisa: Del Cerro.Montobbio E (1995) La Identidad Dificil. Barçelona: Masson.

Montobbio E (1995) El Viaje del Senor Down al Mundo de los Adultos. Barçelona: Masson.

Montobbio E, Grondona ML (eds) (1994). La Casa Senza Specchi: Quale Identita per l'Inatteso? Torino: Omega.

Chapter 4
Sexuality and Individuals with Down Syndrome

DON C VAN DYKE, DIANNE M MCBRIEN, SIRAJ U SIDDIQI AND MARIO C PETERSEN

Sexuality

The development of a healthy sexual identity is a lifelong process, with each life phase presenting a particular task. Infants and toddlers face the tasks of developing trust and personal autonomy. Young children face the tasks of development of self, intimacy, and physical closeness and with later childhood comes the need to master the concepts of modesty and privacy (Grant 1995; Haka-Ikse and Mian 1993). For the adolescent, significant issues include masturbation, personal safety, and relationships (Grant 1995; Haka-Ikse and Mian 1993; Smith 1995).

Unfortunately, the sexuality of mentally disabled people has historically been ignored or denied (Carmody 1996). Prior to the last decade, most of this population was housed in large, sex-segregated institutions with few opportunities to socialize. Society in the past has tended to view mentally disabled people as asexual or, if they appear overly affectionate, hypersexual (Carmody 1996). However, personal relationships and sexuality are essential to the normal development of all adults, including those adults both with and without physical and/or mental disabilities (Smith 1995). While some mentally disabled individuals may not be able to participate in the most typical societal relationship - marriage with children - they can still participate in interpersonal relationships in meaningful ways. The healthy expression of sexuality need not require sexual intercourse, and can take a broad range of forms including close friendship, physical closeness, and nongenital contact.

This presentation reviews the current literature on sexuality and related issues in people with Down syndrome. Specific topics covered include sex education, abuse, reproductive health issues, contraception, and marriage. Because of an almost complete lack of data, the issues of homosexuality, transsexuality, prostitution, and sexual dysfunction in this population will not be discussed.

Sex education

An increasing body of literature and a growing dialogue exist regarding sexuality and sexual expression for individuals with mental disabilities (Ames 1991; Parker and Abramson 1995). Unfortunately, these have not been combined with an equal growth in appropriate programmes for sex education, parent education, the development of support systems, and mechanisms for guidance to help ensure appropriate opportunities and meaningful sexual and personal relationships (Parker and Abramson 1995; Shepperdson 1995)

Comprehensive sex education that includes training in personal and emotional safety as well as in relationship issues should be a standard part of the educational programme for all individuals with Down syndrome (Edwards 1997). Although many such curricula already exist, they are often limited to the discussion of abstinence, contraception, and safe sex. While prevention of disease and unwanted pregnancy is important, it is also vital that such programmes address appropriate social behaviours, privacy issues, relationships, and personal values (Pueschel 1996, 1997).

The current educational trend is towards open and early sex education in the classroom and in the family. Whether sexual information should be provided by the family or by the school, and which moral traditions and values should be reflected in the curriculum, are both topics of continuing debate. In any case, school-based sex education programmes should include all students with developmental disabilities. Since individuals with Down syndrome have a wide range of cognitive levels, learning styles, living and work arrangements, and health issues, such programmes require an individualized approach (Pueschel 1996; Van Dyke et al. 1995).

One popular curriculum in this subject area is the Circles Concept curriculum (Walker-Hirsch and Champagne 1992). This method uses a set of large, brightly coloured concentric circles as a paradigm of physical and emotional distance. Each coloured circle represents a level of physical and emotional intimacy. As students stand in each circle, they learn the appropriate level of physical contact for each level of emotional intimacy.

An eight-week course of sex education has been developed by Elkins (1997) and is outlined in Appendix 4.1. It includes the Circles Concept as well as other materials.

For those individuals with severe cognitive or sensory deficits, the 'good touch/bad touch-model' should be considered (Van Dyke et al. 1995). This concept can be used to teach self-protection skills (Haseltine and Miltenberger 1990) and is often used in elementary schools to teach children to recognize sexually abusive behaviour (Monat-Haller 1992).

Reproduction/pregnancy

Approximately 70 per cent of women with Down syndrome are estimated to be fertile (Hsiang et al. 1987; Tricomi et al. 1964). Studies by Scola of basal body temperature curves suggest that ovulation occurs in approximately 89 per cent of women with Down syndrome (Scola and Pueschel 1992). Hsiang et al. demonstrated elevated luteinizing hormone (LH) and follicle-stimulating hormone (FSH) levels in a group of postpubertal females with Down syndrome, suggesting some degree of primary ovarian dysfunction (Hsiang et al. 1987). Pregnancies have been documented in this population with both Rani et al. and Bovicelli et al. reporting pregnancies in more than 30 women with Down syndrome, resulting in liveborn infants both chromosomally normal and with trisomy 21 (Bovicelli et al. 1982; Rani et al. 1990). This number probably represents only a fraction of actual conceptions.

Pregnancy may put a woman with Down syndrome at high medical risk. Smaller maternal size, potential medical issues common in this population such as cardiac malformation, thyroid dysfunction and seizures, and potential problems understanding and adhering to prenatal care regimens all represent risks for both mother and foetus. Pregnant women with Down syndrome should be referred to a high-risk obstetric facility with teams of professionals experienced in caring for developmentally disabled women and their pregnancies.

Birth control

In the United States, an estimated one million pregnancies occur per year in young females between the ages of 15 and 19 years; about half of these are brought to term (Spitz et al. 1993). It has been estimated that nearly half of all female high school students are sexually active (Gold 1995). The level of sexual activity of females with Down syndrome is unknown, but is thought to be low. In a study by Goldstein (1988) of 15 female adolescents with Down syndrome and 33 age and sex-matched controls, 13 of the girls with Down syndrome had not had sexual intercourse while no information was available on the remaining 2. Nine of the 33 controls (27%) were sexually active.

No forms of contraception are totally contraindicated for women with Down syndrome (Elkins 1997; Schwab 1992). Methods of contraception available to women include abstinence, surgical sterilization, hormonal therapy including Depo-Provera, Norplant, and oral contraceptives, the intrauterine device (Dalkon shield), cervical cap, diaphragm, spermicidal foams and gels, and female condoms (Doty 1995; Elkins 1990; Laros 1993; Lawson and Elkins 1997). The most frequently selected methods include abstinence and, because of their relative ease, the hormonal methods (Lawson and Elkins 1997; Van Dyke et al. 1995). The major contraindications to hormonal therapy in this population are the same for women with

Down syndrome as for women in the general population: dysfunctional uterine bleeding, history of breast cancer, liver disease, and ongoing or history of thromboembolic disease (Heaton 1995). Relative contraindications particular to women with Down syndrome include abnormal thyroid function; chronic treatment with anticonvulsants, systemic antibiotics, or antifungal medications; and cardiac abnormalities, in particular congenital heart disease (Heaton 1995; Van Dyke et al. 1995).

Surgical contraceptive procedures include laparoscopic tubal ligation, total abdominal hysterectomy, and endometrial ablation (Laros 1993; Lawson and Elkins 1997; Van Dyke et al. 1995). Surgical sterilization of mentally disabled women remains a controversial subject (American College of Obstetrics and Gynecology 1988; Heaton 1995; Patterson-Keels et al. 1994, Villanueva 1994). Major parental reasons for considering surgical sterilization are fear of pregnancy from sexual abuse, sexual activity, and contraceptive failure (Patterson-Keels et al. 1994). Such procedures require informed consent and the involvement of patient, parents or legal guardians, guardian ad litem and other legal advocates. Consent in most cases requires review by a human subjects review committee or hospital ethics review board. The process for some parents may be emotionally burdensome and financially draining. Useful resources include the American College of Obstetrics and Gynecologists Committee on Ethics publications or an attorney with experience with disability advocacy issues.

Sexual abuse

As individuals with Down syndrome become more independent and visible members of the community, they become more vulnerable to emotional and sexual abuse (Carmody 1996; Pueschel 1996). The child abuse literature has documented that individuals with mental disabilities are clearly at increased risk for physical, sexual, and emotional abuse (Furey 1994; Schor 1987; Schwab 1992).

Some study groups of mentally retarded individuals have shown incidences of sexual abuse as high as 50 per cent (Elvik et al. 1990; Schor 1987). Sexual abuse is more common in females, and with those with borderline to mild mental retardation. The incidence of abuse decreases as the level of retardation becomes more severe (Elvik et al. 1990; Furey 1994; Schor 1987). Of even greater concern is that many people with mental retardation may be victims of recurrent episodes of sexual abuse (Ammerman et al. 1989; Schor 1987;).

Multiple factors predispose this population to abuse. Social isolation, communication and cognitive problems, and a small peer group all combine to put individuals with mental retardation at increased risk for sexual exploitation and abuse (Schor 1987). The living environment, which can be communal and involve multiple and transient caretakers, compounds the risk (Schor 1987). People with mental disabilities may be quite lonely and grateful for any form of attention; their often strong desire to be 'normal' and anxiety to please may predispose them to tolerate sexual maltreatment (Heaton 1995).

Masturbation

Masturbation is a normal part of self-discovery (Etem and Leventhal 1995; Haka-Ikse and Mian 1993; Monat-Haller 1992;). It may provide gratification in itself or be a prelude to intercourse. In some individuals with mental disability, it may represent self-stimulatory or self-injurious behaviour. Reports of masturbation in males (40%) and females (52%) with Down syndrome demonstrate that this behaviour is not more common in persons with Down syndrome than in the general population (Goldstein 1988; Myers and Pueschel 1991; Rogers and Coleman 1992). Masturbation by the adolescent with Down syndrome may signal an emerging interest in sexuality. This behaviour may be disturbing and uncomfortable for caretakers, parents, and others in the community. If done in public, it may provoke embarrassment and discomfort in others.

Sex education should not focus on stopping masturbation, but on directing the activity towards appropriate times and private places (Edwards 1997). Most individuals with Down syndrome can be taught which times and places are appropriate for this activity. Relieving the discomfort of parents and caregivers may be more difficult, particularly if they view individuals with developmental disabilities as asexual (Edwards 1997).

Female Health Issues in Down Syndrome

Routine gynecological care is not typically provided to women with Down syndrome. In a study by Goldstein (1988) only 7 per cent of females with Down syndrome had ever undergone gynaecological examination, in contrast to 64 per cent of controls (Goldstein 1988). Elkins et al. (1987) report markedly lower usage of reproductive health services by women with Down syndrome.

The timing of menarche in females with Down syndrome is similar to that in the general population (13.6 vs. 13.5 years) (Goldstein 1988). The age of menarche in the United States by 1990 was 12.5 years (Howard 1989). A later study by Scola and Pueschel found a mean menarchal age of 12 years 6 months in this population with a control menarchal age of 12 years 1 month (Scola and Pueschel 1992). Neither precocious nor delayed puberty is a normal finding in women with Down syndrome; both require appropriate evaluation with special attention to thyroid and cardiac status. Goldstein found that the mean duration of both menstrual bleeding and cycle are close to that of women in the general population (Goldstein 1988). Protracted bleeding and other menstrual cycle abnormalities are not normal findings and need evaluation.

With appropriate guidance, many women with Down syndrome can manage their own menstrual hygiene (Kaur et al. 1997a; Scola and Pueschel 1992). In general, if a woman toilets independently, then she may reasonably be expected to perform her own menstrual cares (Kaur et al. 1997b). Educational programmes successful in teaching this form of personal hygiene are concrete and repetitive (Kaur et al. 1997b).

Gynaecological problems

There is little information on rates of breast cancer, reproductive tract cancer, menorrhagia, or leiomyoma in women with Down syndrome (Heaton 1995). McNeeley and Elkins reported in 1989 that 37 of 300 (12%) of women with mental retardation, including many with Down syndrome, required hysterectomy or other uterine surgery. About half of these surgeries were indicated for menorrhagia or symptomatic leiomyoma. Of the 300 cases, only three had malignancies - one uterine and two ovarian cancers (McNeely and Elkins 1989)

Only a few studies document menstrual cycle abnormalities in women with Down syndrome (Heaton 1995). Some data suggests that prolonged flow, a shortened cycle, and irregular bleeding may be more common in women with Down syndrome (Jones and Douglas 1989; Mishell 1987). Menstrual cycle problems in this population should prompt the same evaluations indicated in all women, with particular attention paid to evaluating thyroid function. Dysmenorrhea and premenstrual syndrome are at least as common as in the general population (Heaton 1995; Scola and Pueschel 1992). Since weight gain is a major concern in the older female with Down syndrome, a low-fat meal plan and regular exercise should be an integral part of health care (Sustrova and Pueschel 1997).

Routine gynaecological health maintenance

Routine gynaecological health maintenance for women with Down syndrome is ideally similar to that of all women. Goals of reproductive health care for women in this population are the same as for any woman: screening for breast and reproductive tract disease, treatment of menstrual cycle abnormalities, and, if desired, contraceptive treatment.

An annual mammogram is recommended for all women over 50 years of age (Heaton 1995). In this population, the first mammogram should be approached like the first pelvic examination: slowly and patiently, with much teaching and modelling. A significant family member or caregiver should be present or nearby for support.

A pelvic examination and Pap smear should be performed every one to three years beginning with the first episode of intercourse or the woman's eighteenth year of life, whichever comes first (Brown and Hillard 1996; Heaton 1995). After the baseline exam, women who are not sexually active need the exam repeated every three to five years or as medically indicated.

Women with a history of sexual activity continue to need an annual exam. Because of anxiety about the procedure, some women may benefit from sedation (Brown et al. 1992). Ketamine and midazolam have both been reported as appropriate sedatives for the outpatient setting. Examination under general anaesthesia is also an option, but has the drawbacks of anaesthetic-related risks and high cost (Brown et al. 1992).

For women who for whatever reason are unable to tolerate the procedure with adequate sedation, transabdominal pelvic ultrasound is an acceptable, if more expensive, alternative. Because women with Down syndrome have low rates of cervical cancer but higher rates of ovarian and uterine cancer, transabdominal examinations may actually be of greater utility in this population (Heaton 1995). If the incidence of sexual intercourse rises among women with Down syndrome, the ultrasound may not substitute for a thorough internal examination.

Pelvic examination

Preparation, time, and patience are the keys to a successful pelvic examination. Well in advance of the actual examination, caregivers should discuss the procedure in concrete terms using visual aids; diagrams, full-size pictures, dolls, and videotapes have all been used as educational tools for this concept (Heaton 1995). The pelvic examination should be done separately from other medical visits; so that the procedure is unhurried, it should be scheduled for as much time as possible (Heaton 1995). The presence of a parent or other caregiver should be encouraged. In those women who cannot tolerate speculum examination, a Pap smear can be obtained by locating the cervix with a finger and sliding a long Q-tip over the finger to obtain the sample (Elkins 1990).

Male Health Issues in Down Syndrome

Puberty in males with Down syndrome is similar to that of control males in terms of timing of onset and sequence of development (Pueschel et al. 1985). While some authors find no difference in genital size, other authors have reported a relatively small testicular volume (Arnell et al. 1996; Pueschel et al. 1985).

An increased incidence of genital abnormalities, including cryptorchidism and coronal hypospadias, has been reported in males with Down syndrome (Lang et al. 1986; Smith and Berg 1976). These findings should prompt referral for paediatric urologic evaluation.

Reproductive health issues

Most males with Down syndrome are sterile, with only one documented case of biological fatherhood by a man with Down Syndrome (Rogers and Coleman 1992; Sheridan et al. 1989). The aetiology of male sterility is unknown with many aetiologies proposed, among them abnormalities in sperm structure, count, and motility (Van Dyke et al. 1996).

Condoms are the only contraceptive method available to men; they may not be a practical method for some men with Down syndrome because of cognitive and fine motor problems. The question of vasectomy in this population is usually moot as most of these men are presumed sterile (Heaton 1995).

Routine reproductive health maintenance

Examination of the male genitalia should be part of every routine physical examination (Heaton 1995). Genital abnormalities, and precocious or delayed puberty are indications for appropriate evaluation. Some men with Down syndrome, depending on individual cognitive status and level of personal support, may be able to learn testicular self-examination.

Dating and Marriage

No major articles in the medical or psychology literature discuss dating or marriage by people with Down syndrome. Two young men with Down syndrome, however, did speak eloquently of these issues in their book *Count Us In: Growing Up with Down Syndrome*. Co-authors Jason Levitz and Mitchell Kingsley discuss with keen interest such subjects as 'having a date together, missing girl friends, sexual stuff, and being in love with a girl' (Kingsley and Levitz 1994, pp. 74-82.). At one point, Levitz recalls when a school counsellor helped him to understand appropriate physical boundaries with female students. As this incident illustrates, the social and interpersonal skills needed for dating can be taught. Such instruction should occur as part of a life-skills-based school curriculum, preferably well in advance of any actual dating experience (Fegan et al. 1993).

Little is known about people with Down syndrome who marry. In 1988, Edwards published the results of a survey on marriage in this population. Of 38 married subjects with Down syndrome, all but three were women. None of their spouses had Down syndrome, although many had other developmental disabilities. The author found that most of the couples lived in highly supportive environments, including having family and other advocates nearby (Edwards 1988). A developmentally disabled person's right to marry is a controversial issue. In a few instances, this right has been contested in the courts by family members who wished to block or nullify such unions (Davis 1996).

Some individuals with Down syndrome have keen interest in marriage and family. The two young authors of *Count Us In* discuss their ideas of commitment and marriage in great detail. When asked what makes a good husband, one young man replies, '... you need to be able to understand how important and how you are going to support yourself and your wife

... Part of my future plans is to marry and have a wife, but I need more skills' (Kingsley and Levitz 1994, pp. 101-2).

The issue of marriage in this population often frightens families (Edwards 1997). A series of studies by Shepperdson indicates that while caregivers verbally support the right of developmentally disabled people to have sex and to marry, they generally do not support it for their own children (Shepperdson 1995). While a somewhat more permissive caregiver attitude has emerged in the last two decades, it has not yet been always matched by the educational and counselling services necessary to support stable relationships potentially resulting in marriage (Shepperdson 1995).

Parenting and People with Mental Disabilities

Parenting by people with Down syndrome has not yet been discussed in the literature. This information gap is consistent with a similar lack of data on the social experiences that predate child rearing, such as dating and marriage. As Shepperdson stated in his review, few individuals with Down syndrome have been given the education or freedom that are necessary to support sexual relationships leading to procreation (Shepperdson 1995).

Of all the issues related to sexuality in Down syndrome, the topic of parenting by members of this population is probably the most controversial. The child abuse literature clearly reflects the attitude that parenting is too demanding for individuals with cognitive disabilities (Tymchuk 1992) and that children raised by such parents are at high risk of abuse and neglect. Others view mentally retarded parents more optimistically; these writers reason that parents in this population are aware of their need to seek help and so are potentially more capable than parents with normal intelligence but low socioeconomic or educational status (Nigro 1975).

As previously mentioned, women with Down syndrome are often fertile; their infants have a high incidence of Down syndrome. Many chromosomally normal infants of mothers with Down syndrome have also been reported; these infants may have a higher incidence of major organ malformations. Thus, children born to women with Down syndrome are likely to have special needs, which can exacerbate the normal stresses of parenting. Cognitively normal children without Down syndrome born to such parents with Down syndrome may possibly face the complex family dynamics, as is commonly seen in couples with dwarfism and congenital deafness who produce unaffected children. These couples often fear not that they will have a child like themselves, but they will have a child who is not like them.

Support systems

Physicians, parents, and educators need to provide the individual with Down syndrome with opportunities for learning, for new experiences, for success, and for failures (Smith 1995). These normal developmental needs may sometimes be neglected in the protected environment of home and school. Individuals need to learn daily living skills, appropriate socialization, and group behaviour (Smith 1995). Those individuals in work environments outside of the sheltered workshop need special guidance and support. For those few entering marriage, a supportive network of family and other advocates is important to maintaining the relationship (Edwards 1988).

Working/vocational issues

Work is not only a source of income but also of self-esteem, particularly in American society (Smith 1995). Employment options need not be limited to sheltered workshop settings, and successful placement is possible in a variety of work environments (Smith 1995). For example, several American companies such as McDonald's and Pizza Hut have made the employment of people with developmental disabilities a corporate priority. Learning how to deal with sexual harassment, emotional intimidation, or other similar problems in the work place needs to be part of socialization and vocational preparation during middle and secondary education. Social skills training including sex education, vocational rehabilitation training and work experience all need to be part of the curriculum for students with Down syndrome.

Emotional issues in adults

Placement in a job, however, is only the first step in successful employment; the worker with Down syndrome may need extensive support on the job. A team which includes, at minimum, the individual's employer and a job coach must provide ongoing training, performance monitoring and appropriate supervision. Since individuals with Down syndrome may be at risk for depression and adjustment reactions, the team should strive for a calm, supportive atmosphere in which the employee's emotional status can be monitored (Chicoine et al. 1994; Smith 1995).

Psychiatric disorders are reported in fewer than 25 per cent of children and adolescents with Down syndrome (Myers and Pueschel 1991). Studies show a lower incidence of conduct disorders, neuroses, paranoia, and schizophrenia in people with Down syndrome when compared to control groups with mental retardation of other aetiologies (Collacott et al. 1992; Myers and Pueschel 1991).

Individuals with Down syndrome are, however, at some risk for depression and adjustment reactions sometimes associated with relationships (Chicoine et al. 1994; Myers and Pueschel 1991). Many of these individuals are women in their late twenties and early thirties (Prasher and Hall 1996). Early identification and treatment of these problems are important. Supportive services fostering community integration, social skills, and self-esteem are important preventive measures for depression (Sloper and Turner 1996; Smith 1995).

Acknowledgment

We gratefully acknowledge the editorial assistance of Marilyn Dolezal and Susan Eberly. We are extremely grateful to Dr Thomas E. Elkins, Director, Division of Gynecologic Specialties, Johns Hopkins, Baltimore, Maryland for advice and review of this manuscript.

Appendix 4.1 Sex Education for Individuals with Developmental Disabilities

(An eight-week programme of instruction)

Week #1

Presentation of the positive aspects of who we are as sexual beings.
Bisexuality of society, gender and society.
Similarities and differences of males and females.
Pride in differences.
Gender role differences.
Introduction to female and male anatomy.

Week #2

Private vs. public body parts.

Week #3

Private vs. public behaviours with regard to place, time, and language.
Group vs. single appropriate behaviour.

Week #4, Week #5

Circle drills.

Week #6

Preventing sexual abuse.
Situations using Circle Concept.

Week #7

Test on situations.

Week #8

Discussion on marriage, sex, and contraception.

(From: Elkins, personal communication 1997)

References

American College of Obstetrics and Gynecologists Committee (ACOG) Opinion Committee on Ethics (1988) Sterilization of women who are mentally handicapped. Washington DC: ACOG, No. 63.

Ames T (1991) Guideline for providing sexuality-related services to severely and profoundly retarded individuals: The challenge for the nineteen nineties. Sexuality and Disability 9: 113-22.

Ammerman RT, Van Hasselt VB, Hersen M, McGonigle JJ, Lubetsky MJ (1989) Abuse and neglect in psychiatrically hospitalized multihandicapped children. Child Abuse and Neglect, 13: 335-43.

Arnell H, Gustafsson J, Ivarsson SA, Anneren G (1996) Growth and pubertal development in Down syndrome. Acta Paediatrica 85, 9: 1102-6.

Bovicelli L, Orsini LF, Rizzo N, Montacuti V, Bocchetta M (1982) Reproduction in Down syndrome. Obstetrics and Gynecology 59: 13S-17S.

Brown D, Rosen D, Elkins TE (1992) Sedating women with mental retardation for routine gynecologic examination: an ethical analysis. The Journal of Clinical Ethics 3, 1: 68-75.

Brown RT, Hillard P (1996) Opinions in pediatric and adolescent gynecology. Journal of Pediatric and Adolescent Gynecology 9: 45-6.

Carmody MA (1996) Planning a sexuality education curriculum. Active treatment solutions. Washington: Monaco & Associates.

Chicoine B, McGuire D, Hebein S, Gilly D (1994) Development of a clinic for adults with Down syndrome. Mental Retardation 32: 100-6.

Collacott RA, Cooper SA, McGrother C (1992) Differential rates of psychiatric disorders in adults with Down's syndrome compared with other mentally handicapped adults. British Journal of Psychiatry 161: 671-4.

Davis C (1996) Couple with Down syndrome wins fight to stay married. News & Notes of Down Syndrome/Aim High! 7, 3: 15.

Doty S (1995) Health care in adult life and aging. In Redfern DE (ed) Caring for Individuals with Down Syndrome and their Families (Report of the third Ross Round Table on Critical Issues in Family Medicine). Columbus, Ohio: Ross Products Division. pp. 37-44.

Edwards JP (1988) Sexuality, marriage, and parenting for persons with Down syndrome. In Pueschel SM (ed) The Young Person with Down Syndrome. Baltimore, MD: Brookes. pp. 187-204.

Edwards JP (1997) Growing into a social-sexual being. In Pueschel SM, Sustrova M (eds), Adolescents with Down Syndrome. Baltimore, MD: Brookes. pp. 59-69.

Elkins, TE (1990) Gynecologic care. In Pueschel SM, Pueschel JK (eds), Biomedical Concerns in Persons with Down Syndrome. Baltimore, MD: Brookes. pp. 131-46.

Elkins TE (1997) Sex education programme for individuals with developmental disabilities (Personal communication).

Elkins TE, Spinnado J, Muram D (1987) Sexuality and family interaction in Down syndrome: parental report. Journal of Psychosomatic Obstetrics and Gynecology 6: 81-5.

Elvik SL, Berkowitz CD, Nicholas E, Lipman JL, Inkelis SH (1990) Sexual abuse in the developmentally disabled: dilemmas of diagnosis. Child Abuse and Neglect 14: 497-502.

Etem I, Leventhal JM (1995) Masturbation. In Parker S, Zuckerman B (eds) Behavioral and Developmental Pediatrics. Boston: Little Brown. pp. 200-2.

Fegan L, Rauch A, McCarthy W (1993) Sexuality and People with Intellectual Disability. Baltimore, MD: Brookes.

Furey EM (1994) Sexual abuse of adults with mental retardation: who and where. Mental Retardation 32: 173-80.

Gold MA (1995) New Progestin oral contraceptives and the female condom. Pediatric Annals 24, 4: 211-16.

Goldstein H (1988) Menarche, menstruation, sexual relations and contraception of adolescent females with Down syndrome. European Journal of Obstetrics and Gynecology and Reproductive Biology 27: 343-49.

Grant L (1995) Sex and the adolescent. In Parker S, Zuckerman B (eds) Behavioral and Developmental Pediatrics. Boston: Little Brown. pp. 269-77

Haka-Ikse K, Mian, M (1993) Sexuality in children. Pediatrics in Review 14, 10: 401-7.

Haseltine B, Miltenberger RG (1990) Teaching self-protection skills to persons with mental retardation. American Journal of Mental Retardation 95: 188-97.

Heaton CJ (1995). Providing reproductive health services to persons with Down syndrome and other mental retardation. In Redfern DE (ed) Caring for Individuals with Down Syndrome and their Families (Report of the third Ross Round Table on Critical Issues in Family Medicine). Columbus, Ohio: Ross Products Division. pp 82-94.

Howard CP (1989) Endocrinology of puberty. In Hoffmann A, Greydanus D (eds) Adolescent Medicine, 2nd edn. Norwalk, Connecticut: Appleton & Lange. p. 1.

Hsiang YH, Berkovitz GD, Bland GL, Migeon CJ, Warren, AC (1987) Gonadal function in patients with Down syndrome. American Journal of Medical Genetics 27: 449-56.

Jones K, Douglas J (1989) Gynecologic problems. In Rubin I, Crocker A (eds) Developmental Disabilities: Delivery of Medical Care for Children and Adults. Boston: Lea & Febiger. pp. 276-81.

Kaur H, Butler J, Trumble S (1997a) Options for menstrual management. Menstrual Management. World Wide Web (http://www.nas.com/downsyn/staff.html). Boxhill: Australia. pp. 1-11

Kaur H, Butler J, Trumble S (1997b) Menstrual management and women with an intellectual disability: A guide for general practitioners. Menstrual Management. World Wide Web (http://www.nas.com/downsyn/mennman.html). Boxhill: Australia. p. 1-9.

Kingsley J, Levitz M (1994) Count Us In. Growing Up with Down Syndrome. Orlando, FL: Harcourt Brace.

Lang DJ, Van Dyke DC, Heide F, Lowe PL (1986) Hypospadias and urethral abnormalities in Down syndrome. Clinical Pediatrics 26: 40-2.

Laros A (1993) Adolescent Gynecology (Presentation at the University of Iowa Hospitals and Clinics). Iowa City: Iowa.

Lawson JD, Elkins TE (1997) Gynecologic concerns. In Pueschel SM, Sustrova M (eds) Adolescents with Down Syndrome. Baltimore, MD: Brookes. pp. 39-46.

McNeeley SG, Elkins TE (1989) Gynecologic surgery and surgical morbidity in mentally handicapped women. Obstetric and Gynecology 74: 155-8.

Mishell, D (1987) Abnormal uterine bleeding. In Droegemueller W, Herbst A, Mischel D, Stenchever M (eds) Comprehensive Gynecology. St Louis, MO: CV Mosby. pp. 965-93.

Monat-Haller RK (1992) Understanding and Expressing Sexuality. Baltimore, MD: Brookes.

Myers BA, Pueschel SM (1991) Psychiatric disorders in a population with Down syndrome. Journal of Nervous and Mental Disease 179: 609-13.

Nigro G (1975) Sexuality in the handicapped: Some observation on human needs and attitudes. Rehabilitation Literature 36: 202-5.

Parker T, Abramson PR (1995) The law hath not been dead: Protecting adults with mental retardation from sexual abuse and violation of their sexual freedom. Mental Retardation 33, 4: 257-63.

Patterson-Keels L, Quint E, Brown D, Larson D, Elkins TE (1994). Family views on sterilization for their mentally retarded children. Journal of Reproductive Medicine 39, 9: 701-6.

Prasher VP, Hall W (1996) Short-term prognosis of depression in adults with Down's syndrome: Association with thyroid status and effects on adaptive behavior. Journal of Intellectual Disability Research 40, 1: 32-8.

Pueschel SM (1996) Young people with Down syndrome: Transition from childhood to adulthood. Mental Retardation and Developmental Disabilities Research Reviews 2: 90-5.

Pueschel SM (1997) Adolescent development and sexual maturation. In Pueschel SM, Sustrova M (eds) Adolescents with Down Syndrome. Baltimore, MD: Brookes. pp. 35-8.

Pueschel SM, Orson JM, Boylan JM, Pezzullo JC (1985) Adolescent development in males with Down syndrome. American Journal of Diseases of Children 139: 236-9.

Rani AS, Jyothi A, Reddy PP, Reddy OS (1990) Reproduction in Down syndrome. International Journal of Gynecology and Obstetrics 31: 81-6.

Rogers PT, Coleman M (1992) Medical Care in Down Syndrome: A Preventive Medicine Approach. New York: Marcel Dekker.

Schor DP (1987) Sex and sexual abuse in developmentally disabled adolescents. Seminars in Adolescent Medicine 3: 1-7.

Scola PS, Pueschel SM (1992) Menstrual cycles and basal body temperature curves in women with Down syndrome. Obstetrics and Gynecology 79: 91-4.

Schwab WE (1992) Sexuality and community living. In Lott I, McCoy E (eds) Down Syndrome: Advances in Medical Care. New York: Wiley-Liss. pp. 159-66.

Shepperdson B (1995) The control of sexuality in young people with Down's syndrome. Child: Care, Health & Development 21, 5: 333-49.

Sheridan R, Lierena J, Natkins S, Debenham P (1989) Fertility in a male with trisomy 21. Journal of Medical Genetics 26: 294-8.

Sloper P, Turner, S (1996) Progress in social-independent functioning of young people with Down's syndrome. Journal of Intellectual Disability Research 40, 1: 39-48.

Smith DS (1995) The family practitioner as advocate and advocate stimulator. In Redfern DE (ed) Caring for Individuals with Down Syndrome and their Families (Report of the third Ross Round Table on Critical Issues in Family Medicine). Columbus, OH: Ross Products Division. pp. 64-71.

Smith GR, Berg JM (1976) Down's Anomaly. New York: Churchill-Livingstone.

Spitz AM, Ventura SJ, Koonin LM (1993) Surveillance for pregnancy and birth rates among teenagers by state. (United States 1980 and 1990). Atlanta, Georgia: CDC Surveillance Summaries. MMWR, 42, 1-27.

Sustrova M, Pueschel SM (1997) Nutritional Concerns. In Pueschel SM, Sustrova M (eds), Adolescents with Down Syndrome. Baltimore, MD: Brookes. pp. 17-25.

Tricomi V, Valenti C, Hall JE (1964) Ovulatory patterns in Down's syndrome. American Journal of Obstetrics and Gynecology 89: 651-6.

Tymchuk AJ (1992). Predicting adequacy of parenting by people with mental retardation. Child Abuse and Neglect 16, 165-78.

Van Dyke DC, McBrien DM, Mattheis PJ (1996) Psychosexual behavior, sexuality and management issues in individuals with Down's syndrome. In Rondal JA, Perera J, Nadel L, Comblain A (eds) Down's Syndrome. London: Whurr. pp. 191-203.

Van Dyke DC, McBrien DM, Sherbondy A (1995) Issues of sexuality in Down syndrome. Down's Syndrome: Research and Practice 3, 2: 65-9.

Villanueva AS (1994) Esterilización: Protección o Discriminación. Down, 6-7.

Walker-Hirsch L, Champagne MP (1992) Circles III: Safer ways. In Crocker AC, Cohen HJ, Kastner TA (eds), HIV Infection and Developmental Disabilities. Baltimore, MD: Brookes. pp. 147-58.

PART 3
EDUCATION

Chapter 5
Developmental and Systems Linkages in Early Intervention for Children with Down Syndrome

MICHAEL J GURALNICK

The purpose of this chapter is to emphasize the correspondence between a general developmental approach to child development and the system of early intervention programmes for children with Down syndrome. Of course, the value of a developmental perspective in understanding children with Down syndrome has been thoughtfully articulated for many developmental domains and developmental contexts (see Cicchetti and Beeghly 1990). These analyses reveal that a general developmental framework can accommodate most empirical findings. However, there remain concerns that specific and to some extent unique developmental patterns exhibited by children with Down syndrome have not been adequately appreciated (Gibson 1991; Spiker and Hopmann 1997). These differences become highlighted in the context of early intervention programmes, as clinicians are often faced with the need to design practical strategies that do not, on the surface, seem compatible with a developmental framework.

To examine this issue I will first present a general developmental model and link it to well-established short-term early intervention benefits for children with Down syndrome. Central to the developmental model are the notions of proximal family patterns of interaction which mediate more distal family characteristics to influence child developmental outcomes. It is further suggested that these pathways of influence are applicable to all families, irrespective of the child's developmental status. Another pathway of this model consists of unique sets of 'stressors' created by a child's disability. It is the effect of these stressors and their interaction with other possible stressors associated with family characteristics that provide the basis for accommodating to the uniqueness of children with Down syndrome within a larger developmental framework. Addressing these stressors also provides the conceptual and practical linkage to the early intervention system. Considered in this chapter as well are ways in which this framework can help promote longer-term effects of early intervention for children with Down syndrome, with an emphasis on incorporating new developmental findings into early intervention programmes.

Developmental Framework

Figure 5.1 illustrates the major components of the developmental model. The purpose here is to organize and account for the salient *experiential factors* governing child developmental outcomes. The model attempts to accommodate children with a wide range of risk and disability conditions (see Guralnick 1997b, 1998 for details), and has therefore relied upon diverse developmental approaches including Belsky's parenting model (Belsky 1984), Sameroff's transactional model (Sameroff 1993), Ramey's biosocial model (Ramey et al. 1992), Dunst's social support model (Dunst 1985), and Bronfenbrenner's (1979) ecological model.

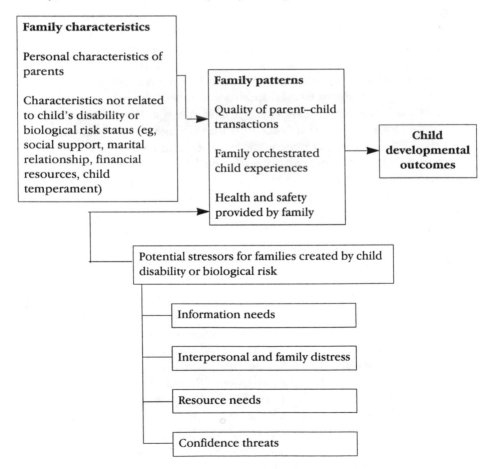

Figure 5.1 Factors influencing developmental outcomes for children.
Source: Guralnick 1997b. Reprinted by permission.

Sufficient evidence is available to suggest that at least three primary and proximal patterns of *family interaction* substantially contribute to child developmental outcomes. First, the quality of parent-child transactions has been most frequently studied and directly linked to child outcomes through various parent-child transaction constructs such as responsivity, sensitivity, scaffolding, and engaging in nonintrusive, affectively warm, and discourse-based exchanges. These well-defined constructs can be readily measured and have been linked to both general and specific forms of child outcome (eg, Baumrind 1993; Clarke-Stewart 1988; Landry et al. 1997; Wachs 1992). Second, experiences families provide and orchestrate for their children, such as the provision of developmentally appropriate and stimulating toys in the home, organizing social interactions with adults and children as part of the parents' social networks, or through the quality of alternative child care options selected, all constitute important experiences linked to child outcomes (eg, Wachs and Gruen 1982). General arrangements for educational, recreational, or special developmental experiences to take advantage of or accommodate their child's unique interests and needs also constitute important family-orchestrated child experiences that influence child developmental outcomes (eg, NICHD Study of Early Child Care 1997; Parke and Ladd 1992). Third, family patterns of interaction that regulate the health and safety of the child, such as nutrition (Gorman 1995), correspond closely to child outcomes.

In turn, the model indicates (see Figure 5.1) that these three proximal patterns of interaction are governed by a set of *family characteristics*. These include personal characteristics of the parents such as intergenerational and culturally transmitted attitudes and beliefs about child rearing, parental mental health, and parents' intellectual abilities. Of importance, should any of these family characteristics not be optimal, they can adversely affect child developmental outcomes (Cicchetti and Toth 1995; Crowell and Feldman 1988; Feldman 1997; Murphey 1992). Moreover, if these more distal, nonoptimal family characteristics are evident, it is suggested that the pathways of influence are mediated by the three family patterns of interaction. In essence, these family patterns are 'stressed' by adverse family characteristics in the sense that they create the basis for nonoptimal family interaction patterns. Risk factors is another term often applied to these stressors.

In many instances, these stressors are longstanding, such as those associated with personal characteristics of the parents. Other family characteristics that can influence family interaction patterns may vary more with external circumstances, and therefore be more amenable to change. In particular, these include failure to establish adequate social supports (Cochran and Brassard 1979; Melson et al. 1993), stressful marital relationships (Emery and Kitzmann 1995), and limited financial resources (Duncan et al. 1994; McLoyd 1990); all of which have been associated with nonoptimal child developmental outcomes. Moreover, individual child characteristics (eg, temperament), unrelated to a child's risk or disability status, also can create stressful parent-child transactions (Lee and Bates 1985; Sameroff 1993).

Stressors Related to A Child's Disability

When a child is born with Down syndrome, a set of additional potential stressors capable of perturbing family patterns of interaction come into play. These stressors can be organized into four types (see Figure 5.1). First, stressors emerge in the form of information needs. Issues related to the health of their child (Cooley and Graham 1991; Hayes and Batshaw 1993), emerging discrepancies between receptive and expressive language (Fowler 1990; Rondal 1996), attentional difficulties (eg, Kasari et al. 1995), or lack of correspondence between child and parent affective expressions (Knieps et al. 1994), can all potentially adversely affect family patterns of interaction. Similarly, parents of children with Down syndrome may experience difficulties organizing playgroups with peers for their children (Guralnick 1997a; Stoneman 1993) and, like other families of children with disabilities, must continuously consider questions about the value of specific therapeutic services and how to gain access to the best professionals and programmes (see Sontag and Schacht 1994). Different issues, of course, emerge as development proceeds, but all have the potential to perturb optimal family interaction patterns.

Interpersonal and family distress, the second type of potential stressor, can also adversely influence family interaction patterns. The birth of a child with a disability results in an intensely emotional experience, often creating reassessments of expectations and goals within the family (eg, Hodapp et al. 1992) and adjustments in family roles and routines (Barnett and Boyce 1995). Many families of children with disabilities do indeed adapt extremely well (eg, Trute and Hauch 1988), and this is certainly true for families of children with Down syndrome. Nevertheless, the same forces that create distress for children with disabilities in general seem to operate for families of children with Down syndrome (Cahill and Glidden 1996). In fact, affective distress engendered by the parenting process itself has been well documented for families of children with Down syndrome (Atkinson et al. 1995), and distress to varying degrees is likely to recur as the child moves through different developmental stages and transition points (Wikler 1986). Finally, the risk of social isolation for families remains, as even contemporary Western societies have failed to discard the all-too-pervasive negative attitudes toward people with disabilities and their families (see Stoneman 1993).

The third type of potential stressor that can disrupt family interaction patterns concerns unusual resource needs that frequently arise as a consequence of having a child with Down syndrome. As noted, the usual routines of a family are often disrupted and can affect the quality of caregiving (Beckman 1983; Dyson 1993). Locating and sometimes coordinating services is a responsibility often assumed by families, thereby creating additional demands on their time and resources (Rubin and Quinn-Curran 1985). Financial concerns may mount as well as a consequence of increased health care and related expenses. In fact, caregiving responsibilities may limit mothers' opportunities for out-of-home work and the income it generates (Barnett and Boyce 1995; Kelly and Booth 1997).

Finally, taken together, these three sources of stressors can ultimately undermine parental confidence in their ability to provide appropriate caregiving. This insidious process can have long-term negative consequences as families are certain to encounter challenge after challenge as their child develops (see Cooley 1994).

Impact of Stressors on Development

Should these four types of potential stressors actually have an effect, the model suggests that they do so by adversely influencing one or more of the three family interaction patterns. Available evidence indicates that in the absence of early intervention, these stressful influences do, in fact, manifest themselves for families of children with Down syndrome. In particular, a consistent finding is a general decline in intellectual development that occurs across the first five years of life (Carr 1970; Connolly 1978; Melyn and White 1973; Morgan 1979). The order of magnitude of this decline is approximately .50-.75 SD (8-12 IQ points) and does not appear to be related to a cohort effect, although the relatively steep decline across the first 18 months of life may well be due, in part, to an increasingly larger proportion of test items devoted to cognitive and language development (Guralnick and Bricker 1987; Neser et al. 1989). However, the continuing decline may well be attributed to experiential factors; ie, to stressors linked to family interaction patterns.

It is important to note that considerable individual differences exist with regard to the extent to which stressors actually produce an adverse impact. The severity of the stressors themselves will certainly account for some of that variability. However, as Figure 5.1 indicates, family interaction patterns are a joint function of stressors due to a child's disability and family characteristics. As such, even significant child disability-related stressors may be able to be mitigated by family resources or related protective factors. The coping capacities of families should not be underemphasized. On the other hand, family characteristics can produce stressors of their own, interacting with stressors associated with a child's disability and risk status to create substantial perturbations in family interaction patterns. Of note, in the United States approximately one-third of families of children with disabilities live at or below generally accepted definitions for low income (Bowe 1995). This 'double vulnerability' can have very damaging effects on child development (see Bradley et al. 1994).

The Early Intervention System

If this developmental model is correct, then effective early intervention programmes should be organized to respond to these stressors. In fact, as suggested in Figure 5.2, analyses of existing components of early intervention programmes indicate that programmes do indeed appear to be structured in that manner. Three general components can be readily identified. First, resource supports are provided in the form of organizing and coordinating the many-faceted aspects of health, educational, and social services. Service coordination is always a challenge, yet a coherent, comprehensive set of services and supports is critical for successful early intervention (Guralnick, 1998). In addition, as noted earlier, many families require supplemental supports such as financial assistance and respite care.

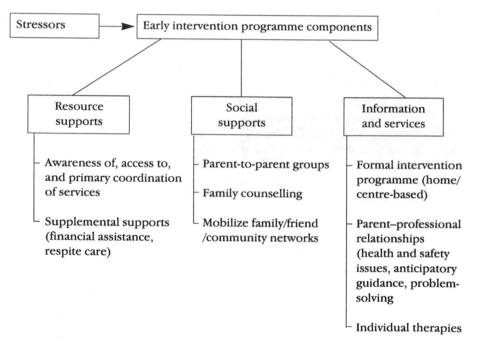

Figure 5.2 Components of early intervention programmes as a response to stressors. Source: Guralnick 1997b. Reprinted by permission.

Social supports provided by numerous and well-established parent organizations, in particular, have emerged as a vital component of the early intervention system (Santelli et al. 1995). These and more specific family counselling services can have a significant positive impact on interpersonal and family distress and provide families with important information in a timely and sensitive manner.

Perhaps the most visible component of the early intervention system is that concerning information and services. Children participate in some combination of home- and/or centre-based programmes as part of the formal aspects of the early intervention system. In these programmes, children experience clinician-organized or -directed interventions, usually guided by specific curricula (Bailey 1997; Bruder 1997). The structure and direction provided by these diverse curricula appear to be essential for their effectiveness (Shonkoff and Hauser-Cram 1987). Special therapeutic services are usually provided in the context of these more formal programmes, although parents often build important relationships with professionals who provide therapeutic services outside of this context. These partnerships can form a vital professional support network that can help resolve many parental dilemmas and serve as resources for anticipatory guidance and general approaches to problem-solving. It is important to note that even with therapeutic services that are integrated in the formal intervention programmes, the total amount of such services tends to be small. For infants and toddlers with Down syndrome in the United States, the average amount of time spent in these formal intervention programmes is approximately seven hours per month. However, as reflected in Figure 5.2, it is the totality of the supports and services that must be considered in both the design and evaluation of early intervention programmes. Together, these three components can have the effect of increasing parental confidence and competence, characteristics so essential for effective outcomes (see Cooley 1994).

Short-term effectiveness

When comprehensive early intervention programmes are provided to children with Down syndrome and their families, a substantial positive effect is obtained. In fact, when children are enrolled during the first year of life, much of the decline in intellectual development described earlier that occurs in the absence of early intervention can be minimized substantially or eliminated entirely while children are enrolled in programmes (Berry et al. 1984; Schnell 1984; Sharav and Shlomo 1986; Woods et al. 1984). Of course, significant delays are still present, but the reductions in decline constitute an important accomplishment. Presumably, resource supports, social supports, and information and services are appropriately matched to individual child and family needs in well-designed early intervention programmes so that potential stressors influencing family interaction patterns are minimized.

Long-term effectiveness

Despite consistent evidence supporting the immediate and short-term effectiveness of early intervention for children with Down syndrome, concerns exist with regard to the impact of these programmes on children's long-term development. After all, the expectation that long-term effects will result and the corresponding justification for a substantial investment in the early years have a firm basis in developmental psychology and developmental neurobiology (Anastasiow 1990; Guralnick and Bennett 1987; Rutter 1980). Yet, as Gibson and Harris (1988) point out, the fact is that virtually no evidence is available to indicate that children with Down syndrome do better in the long-term as a consequence of participation in early intervention programmes. Certainly the quality of the post-early intervention environment is critical, and has yet to be taken fully into account. For the most part, however, adequate studies have simply not been carried out to evaluate this issue.

Despite this state-of-affairs, except in countries with poorly developed early intervention systems, it is unlikely for practical reasons that well-designed clinical trials of the long-term effectiveness of early intervention for children with Down syndrome will be possible. This is certainly true for straightforward comparisons of children receiving or not receiving early intervention services.

Nevertheless, the question of long-term effectiveness has been addressed for related populations of children with disabilities and those at risk for developmental delays, and can provide useful information for programmes for children with Down syndrome. A recent analysis conducted by Guralnick (1998) has revealed that sustained long-term effects can be reliably obtained if early intervention programmes are comprehensive, time intensive, or of extended duration (eg, extend throughout the child's first five years of life), and are available to help families through important transition points. It is likely that most, if not all, of these same features are relevant to the early intervention system serving children with Down syndrome. Of importance, a number of hypotheses about long-term effectiveness can be generated and tested to determine the extent to which these and other factors can influence long-term effectiveness of early intervention. Clinical trials comparing different intensities of intervention, for example, can materially contribute to evaluating long-term effectiveness yet continue to provide needed services to children and families.

Programme improvements

Ongoing developmental research further suggests that existing early intervention programmes can become even more effective by considering recent findings. In essence, research is now focusing on the identification of subgroups of families whose family interaction patterns do not appear to be optimal in specific ways. If properly identified, special targeted interventions could be provided and the variability in early intervention outcomes further reduced. This process of refinement of the early intervention system may have implications for both short- and long-term effectiveness.

For example, recent evidence suggests that the ability of parents of children with Down syndrome to sustain their attention to child-selected toys is related to more advanced child receptive language (Harris et al.1996). Presumably, this increased level of joint attention to an object of the child's interest allows the child to allocate adequate cognitive resources to the receptive language features of the context. Again, this interaction pattern is apparent only for some parents of children with Down syndrome. Similarly, research continues to suggest that there exists a small subgroup of parents of children with Down syndrome who tend to adopt a more 'performance-oriented' approach when interacting with their child (see Mahoney and Powell 1988; Mahoney et al. 1992; Spiker and Hopmann 1997). This highly directive pattern is not consistent with optimally promoting children's cognitive development, as it limits opportunities for more discourse-based, child-initiated, and challenging exchanges.

Other aspects of the relationship between parents and their children with Down syndrome can be affected as well, with potentially widespread developmental implications. In particular, recent findings suggest that an avoidance coping style adopted by some parents of children with Down syndrome can reduce sensitivity to their child's cues (Atkinson et al. 1995). Other work has demonstrated that some parents of children with Down syndrome direct fewer internal state words related to both emotion and cognition to their children than do parents of typically developing children (Tingley et al. 1994). These differences in parents' lexicon may have long-term consequences for children's self-regulation of affective and cognitive abilities. Taken together, through continuing research and programmatic efforts to fine-tune early intervention programmes by considering these issues based on emerging developmental research for specific subgroups of families and determining the configuration of programme elements that maximize long-term outcomes, even greater short- and long-term benefits of early intervention for children with Down syndrome are likely to be realized in the future.

Conclusions

The positive short-term effects of early intervention, particularly on the cognitive development of children with Down syndrome, can be well understood within a developmental framework. The concept of stressors that can adversely affect family interaction patterns can be linked to the design of responsive early intervention systems. However, additional research is needed to evaluate the long-term effectiveness and the factors influencing these outcomes. Finally, fine tuning of early intervention programmes to unique parent-child patterns of subgroups of families of children with Down syndrome may be especially beneficial.

References

Anastasiow NJ (1990) Implications of the neurobiological model for early intervention. In Meisels SJ, Shonkoff JP (eds) Handbook of Early Childhood Intervention. Cambridge: Cambridge University Press. pp. 196-216.

Atkinson L, Chisholm V, Dickens S, Scott B, Blackwell J, Tam F, Goldberg S (1995) Cognitive coping, affective distress, and maternal sensitivity: Mothers of children with Down syndrome. Developmental Psychology 31: 668-76.

Bailey DB (1997) Evaluating the effectiveness of curriculum alternatives for infants and preschoolers at high risk. In Guralnick MJ (ed) The Effectiveness of Early Intervention. Baltimore, MD: Brookes. pp. 227-47.

Barnett WS, and Boyce GC (1995) Effects of children with Down syndrome on parents' activities. American Journal on Mental Retardation 100: 115-27.

Baumrind D (1993) The average expectable environment is not good enough: A response to Scarr. Child Development 64: 1299-317.

Beckman PJ (1983) Characteristics of handicapped infants: A study of the relationship between child characteristics and stress as reported by mothers. American Journal of Mental Deficiency 88: 150-6.

Belsky J (1984) The determinants of parenting: A process model. Child Development 55: 83-96.

Berry P, Gunn VP, Andrews RJ (1984) Development of Down's syndrome children from birth to five years. In Berg JM (ed) Perspectives and Progress in Mental Retardation: Vol. 1. Social, Psychological, and Educational Aspects. Baltimore: University Park Press. pp. 167-77.

Bowe FG (1995) Population estimates: Birth-to-5 children with disabilities. The Journal of Special Education 20: 461-71.

Bradley RH, Whiteside L, Mundfrom DJ, Casey PH, Kelleher KJ, Pope SK (1994) Early indications of resilience and their relation to experiences in the home environments of low birthweight, premature children living in poverty. Child Development 65: 346-60.

Bronfenbrenner U (1979) The Ecology of Human Development. Cambridge, MA: Harvard University Press.

Bruder MB (1997) The effectiveness of specific educational/developmental curricula for children with established disabilities In Guralnick MJ (ed) The Effectiveness of Early Intervention. Baltimore, MD: Brookes. pp. 523-48.

Cahill BM, Glidden LM (1996) Influence of child diagnosis on family and parental functioning: Down syndrome versus other disabilities. American Journal on Mental Retardation 101: 149-60.

Carr J (1970) Mental and motor development in young mongol children. Journal of Mental Deficiency Research 14: 205.

Cicchetti D, Beeghly M (eds) (1990) Children with Down Syndrome: A Developmental Perspective. Cambridge: Cambridge University Press.

Cicchetti D, Toth SL (1995) Developmental psychopathology and disorders of affect. In Cicchetti D and Cohen DJ (eds) Developmental Psychopathology: Risk, Disorder, and Adaptation, Vol. 2. New York: Wiley. pp. 369-420.

Clarke-Stewart KA (1988) Parents' effects on children's development: A decade of progress? Journal of Applied Developmental Psychology 9: 41-84.

Cochran MM and Brassard JA (1979) Child development and personal social networks. Child Development 50: 601-15.

Connolly JA (1978) Intelligence levels of Down's syndrome children. American Journal of Mental Deficiency 83: 193-6.

Cooley WC (1994) The ecology of support for caregiving families. Commentary. Journal of Developmental and Behavioral Pediatrics 15: 117-9.

Cooley WC, Graham JM (1991) Common syndromes and management issues for primary care physicians. Clinical Pediatrics 30: 233-53.

Crowell JA, Feldman SS (1988) Mothers' internal models of relationships and children's behavioral and developmental status: a study of mother-child interaction. Child Development 59: 1273-85.

Duncan GJ, Brooks-Gunn J, Klebanov PK (1994) Economic deprivation and early childhood development. Child Development 65: 296-318.

Dunst CJ (1985) Rethinking early intervention. Analysis and Intervention in Developmental Disabilities 5: 165-201.

Dyson LL (1993). Response to the presence of a child with disabilities: parental stress and family functioning over time. American Journal on Mental Retardation 98: 207-18.

Emery RE, Kitzmann AM (1995) The child in the family: disruptions in family functions. In Cicchetti D, Cohen DJ (eds) Developmental Psychopathology: Risk, Disorder, and Adaptation Vol. 2. New York: Wiley. pp. 3-31.

Feldman MA (1997) The effectiveness of early intervention for children of parents with mental retardation. In Guralnick MJ (ed) The Effectiveness of Early Intervention. Baltimore, MD: Brookes. pp. 171-91.

Fowler AE (1990) Language abilities in children with Down syndrome: evidence for a specific syntactic delay. In Cicchetti D, Beeghly M (eds) Children with Down Syndrome: A Developmental Perspective. Cambridge: Cambridge University Press. pp. 302-28.

Gibson D (1991) Down syndrome and cognitive enhancement: not like the others. In Marfo K (ed) Early Intervention in Transition: Current Perspectives on Programs for Handicapped Children. New York: Praeger. pp. 61-90.

Gibson D, Harris A (1988) Aggregated early intervention effects for Down's syndrome persons: Patterning and longevity of benefits. Journal of Mental Deficiency Research 32: 1-17.

Gorman KS (1995) Malnutrition and cognitive development: Evidence from experimental/quasi-experimental studies among the mild-to-moderately malnourished. Journal of Nutrition 125: 2239S-2244S.

Guralnick MJ (1997a) The peer social networks of young boys with developmental delays. American Journal on Mental Retardation 101: 595-612.

Guralnick MJ (1997b) Second generation research in the field of early intervention. In Guralnick MJ (ed) The Effectiveness of Early Intervention. Baltimore, MD: Brookes. pp. 3-22.

Guralnick MJ (1998) The effectiveness of early intervention for vulnerable children: A developmental perspective. American Journal on Mental Retardation 102: 319-45.

Guralnick MJ, Bennett FC (1987) A framework for early intervention. In Guralnick MJ, Bennett FC (eds) The Effectiveness of Early Intervention for At-risk and Handicapped Children. New York: Academic Press. pp. 3-29.

Guralnick MJ, Bricker D (1987) The effectiveness of early intervention for children with cognitive and general developmental delays. In Guralnick MJ, Bennett FC (eds) The Effectiveness of Early Intervention for At-risk and Handicapped Children. New York: Academic Press. pp. 115-73.

Harris S, Kasari C, Sigman MD (1996) Joint attention and language gains in children with Down syndrome. American Journal on Mental Retardation 100: 608-19.

Hayes A, Batshaw ML (1993) Down syndrome. Pediatric Clinics of North America 40: 523-35.

Hodapp RM, Dykens EM, Evans DW, Merighi JR (1992) Maternal emotional reactions to young children with different types of handicaps. Journal of Developmental and Behavioral Pediatrics 13: 118-23.

Kasari C, Freeman S, Mundy P, Sigman MD (1995) Attention regulation by children with Down syndrome: Coordinated joint attention and social referencing looks. American Journal on Mental Retardation 100: 128-36.

Kelly JF, Booth CL (1997) Child care for infants at risk and with disabilities: Description and issues in the first 15 months. Poster session presented at the annual meeting of the Society for Research in Child Development. Washington DC.

Knieps LJ, Walden TA, Baxter A (1994) Affective expressions of toddlers with and without Down syndrome in a social referencing context. American Journal on Mental Retardation 99: 301-12.

Landry SH, Smith KE, Miller-Loncar CL, Swank PR (1997) Predicting cognitive-language and social growth curves from early maternal behaviors in children at varying degrees of biological risk. Developmental Psychology 33: 1040-53.

Lee CL, Bates JE (1985) Mother-child interaction at age two years and perceived difficult temperament. Child Development 56: 1314-25.

Mahoney G, Powell A (1988) Modifying parent-child interaction: enhancing the development of handicapped children. Journal of Special Education 22: 82-96.

Mahoney G, Robinson C, Powell A (1992) Focusing on parent-child interaction: the bridge to developmentally appropriate practices. Topics in Early Childhood Special Education 12: 105-20.

McLoyd VC (1990) The impact of economic hardship on black families and children: psychological distress, parenting and socioemotional development. Child Development 61: 311-46.

Melson GF, Ladd GW, Hsu H-C (1993) Maternal support networks, maternal cognitions, and young children's social and cognitive development. Child Development 64: 1401-17.

Melyn MA, White DT (1973) Mental and developmental milestones of noninstitutionalized Down's syndrome children. Pediatrics 52: 542-5.

Morgan SB (1979) Development and distribution of intellectual and adaptive skills in Down syndrome children: Implications for early intervention. Mental Retardation 17: 247-9.

Murphey DA (1992) Constructing the child: relations between parents' beliefs and child outcomes. Developmental Review 12: 199-232.

Neser PSJ, Molteno CD, Knight GJ (1989) Evaluation of preschool children with Down's syndrome in Cape Town using the Griffiths Scale of Mental Development. Child: Care Health and Development 15: 217-25.

NICHD Study of Early Child Care (1997) Results of NICHD study of early child care. Paper presented at the biennial meeting of the Society for Research in Child Development April 5 1997 Washington, DC.

Parke RD, Ladd GW (eds) (1992) Family-peer relationships: modes of linkage. Hillsdale, NJ: Lawrence Erlbaum.

Ramey CT, Bryant DM, Wasik BH, Sparling JJ, Fendt KH, LaVange LM (1992) Infant health and development program for low birth weight, premature infants: program elements, family participation, and child intelligence. Pediatrics 89: 454-65.

Rondal JA (1996) Oral language in Down's syndrome. In Rondal JA, Perera J, Nadel L, Comblain A (eds), Down's Syndrome: Psychological, Psychobiological and Socio-educational Perspectives. London: Whurr. pp. 99-117.

Rubin S, Quinn-Curran N (1985) Lost, then found: parents' journey through the community service maze. In Seligman M (ed) The Family with a Handicapped Child: Understanding and Treatment. New York: Grune and Stratton. pp. 63-94.

Rutter M (1980) The long-term effects of early experience. Developmental Medicine and Child Neurology 22: 800-15.

Sameroff AJ (1993) Models of development and developmental risk. In Zeanah Jr CH (ed) Handbook of Infant Mental Health. New York: Guilford. pp. 3-13.

Santelli B, Turnbull AP, Marquis JG, Lerner EP (1995) Parent to parent programs: a unique form of mutual support. Infants and Young Children, 8, 2: 48-57.

Schnell R (1984) Psychomotor development. In Peuschel S (ed) The Young Child with Down Syndrome. New York: Human Sciences. pp. 207-226.

Sharav T, Shlomo L (1986) Stimulation of infants with Down syndrome: long-term effects. Mental Retardation 24: 81-6.

Shonkoff JP, Hauser-Cram P (1987) Early intervention for disabled infants and their families: a quantitative analysis. Pediatrics 80: 650-8.

Sontag JC, Schacht R (1994) An ethnic comparison of parent participation and information needs in early intervention. Exceptional Children 60: 422-33.

Spiker D, Hopmann MR (1997) The effectiveness of early intervention for children with Down syndrome. In Guralnick MJ (ed) The Effectiveness of Early Intervention. Baltimore, MD: Brookes. pp. 271-305.

Stoneman Z (1993) The effects of attitude on preschool integration. In Peck CA, Odom SL, Bricker DD (eds) Integrating Young Children with Disabilities into Community Programs. Baltimore: Brookes. pp. 223-48.

Tingley EC, Gleason JB, Hooshyar N (1994). Mothers' lexicon of internal state words in speech to children with Down syndrome and to nonhandicapped children at mealtime. Journal of Communication Disorders 27: 135-55.

Trute B, Hauch C (1988) Building on family strength: a study of families with positive adjustment to the birth of a developmentally disabled child. Journal of Marital and Family Therapy 14: 185-93.

Wachs TD (1992) The Nature of Nurture. Newbury Park, CA: Sage.

Wachs TD, Gruen GE (1982). Early Experience and Human Development. New York: Plenum Press.

Wikler LM (1986) Family stress theory and research on families of children with mental retardation. In Gallagher JJ, Vietze PM (eds) Families of Handicapped Persons. Baltimore, MD: Brookes. pp. 167-95.

Woods PA, Corney MJ, Pryce GJ (1984) Developmental progress of preschool Down's syndrome children receiving a home-advisory service: an interim report. Child: Care, Health and Development 10: 287-99.

Chapter 6
Promoting the Educational Competence of Students with Down Syndrome[1]

JOHN E RYNDERS

For students with Down syndrome and their parents, receiving a strong educational programme - that is, a programme that is appropriately challenging, suitably individualized, adequately supported and reasonably continuous - often involves overcoming barriers. For instance, assessment team members in a school may be reluctant to place a child with Down syndrome in a regular classroom (an option often referred to as 'mainstreaming' or 'inclusionary'), even if assessment outcomes indicate a good chance of success. Why? Possibly because of a longstanding misperception that children with Down syndrome are rarely able to learn academic subjects sufficiently (often referred to as the inability to attain and sustain an 'educable' learning level), but are suited best for learning self-care tasks (a level of attainment often referred to as a 'trainable' level).

The terms 'trainable' and 'educable' used throughout this paper are historic artifacts to some extent. The two terms came into use in the US in the days of self-contained programming as a convenient way for educators to determine a placement or curricular emphasis based on a child's intellectual level (the range of approximately IQ 40 to 55 was generally acknowledged to represent the trainable range, while an IQ range of approximately 55 to 70 was generally accepted as the educable range).

This label/IQ range procedure for making educational decisions, while convenient, has always had limited practical validity. IQ, a score based on

[1] This paper is based in part on an article by John Rynders, Brian Abery, Donna Spiker, Melissa Olive, Christina Sheran and Robert Zajac, titled, 'Improving educational programming for individuals with Down syndrome: engaging the fuller competence' published in Down Syndrome Quarterly, March 1997, Vol. 2, No. 1, pp. 1-11. Development of the article and this paper was partially supported by the University of Minnesota Research and Training Center on Community Integration (NIDRR Cooperative Agreement No. H133B80048). Content and opinions do not necessarily reflect the position or policy of the funding agencies, and no official endorsement should be inferred.

the performance of tasks that were initially chosen to reflect actual schooling activities as little as possible, was paradoxically eventually used as a predictor of school activity achievement outcomes. Nonetheless, I will continue to use the terms 'trainable' and 'educable' throughout this article despite their inherent limitations because they have exerted a strong influence on the placement and programming perceptions of school personnel since 1866, when Dr J Langdon Down offered the first formal description of the condition that continues to bear his name. However, at the end of this article I will suggest alternatives to their continued use.

The purpose of this paper will be to describe the educational accomplishments of 171 students who have Down syndrome, giving particular attention to their academic capabilities since this is such a central issue in educational planning, a point that my associates and I have tried to make on several occasions (Rynders 1995; Rynders and Horrobin 1990; Rynders et al. 1978). Until now, however, a comprehensive and relatively large database from which to explore this point has not been available. It is not our intention, though, to focus attention solely on the academic capability of students with Down syndrome but to take a holistic look at their abilities, including academic, language, cognitive and motor achievements. But first, let us look briefly at portions of Dr Down's description and subsequent educationally related events that appear to have left an indelible impression (often a negative impression) on educators' expectations concerning the learning capacity of individuals with Down syndrome.

An Abbreviated History with a Focus on the Training/Trainable Concept

In 1866, physician John Langdon Down, in providing the first formal description of the condition that bears his name today, used terms that are now considered racist and which have been totally discredited (Ferguson 1995, p. 54). Dr Down, who attempted to classify the various forms of 'feeblemindedness' he had observed, was strongly influenced, as far as we can discern, by Charles Darwin's thoughts on evolution. He concluded that a group of individuals who looked Asiatic to him belonged to the 'Mongolian family'. He then proposed, '... that there can be no doubt that these ethnic features are the result of degeneration' (Down 1866, pp. 260-1). Terminology Down used in his report, including 'degeneration' and 'idiots who arrange themselves around the Mongolian type' cast grave doubt on the overall potential of persons who would eventually come to be known as having a unique chromosomal condition occurring in all racial and ethnic groups, including the populace of Mongolia.

In light of the era of racial elitism in which he lived, it is remarkable that Dr Down did not portray the learning prospects of persons with Down syndrome as hopeless. On the contrary, near the end of his historic article in *Clinical Lectures and Reports* (1866), he offered them a 'back-handed' compliment: 'They are cases which very much repay judicious treatment … the improvement which *training* effects in them is greatly in excess of what would be predicated if one did not know the characteristics of the type' (pp. 261-2, italics added).

The word 'training' in Down's report would figure prominently in a major goal of the residential institutionalization movement: training in unskilled domestic and manual tasks, such as picking farm crops by hand. Between 1866, when Dr Down's report appeared, and the mid-1900s when deinstitutionalization began in earnest, most individuals with Down syndrome in many state institutions such as Northern Wisconsin Colony and *Training* (italics added) School (currently the Northern Wisconsin Center), were trained in unskilled tasks while attending school programmes on institution campuses labelled 'trainable' - that is, if they attended school at all.

Special education services up through the mid-1970s, whether they occurred in training schools within institutions or in public or private schools, were nearly always separated from regular education services to the maximum extent possible. Furthermore, educational access to these self-contained programmes was seldom guaranteed in law to persons with serious developmental disabilities. In fact, a debate raged in the education literature during the late 1950s as to whether students classified as 'trainable' (versus 'educable') should be educated in public schools at all (Cruikshank 1958; Goldberg 1958).

A key opportunity for opening public education programmes to children with Down syndrome came in 1972 in the form of the landmark case: *Pennsylvania Association for Retarded Children v. Commonwealth of Pennsylvania*, (the PARC case). In that litigation, the judge ruled that every child, regardless of type or severity of disability, had a right to a free, appropriate, public programme of education, and that placement in a regular educational setting was preferable to placement in a special education setting. The PARC case led to the passage of PL 94-142, the Education for All Handicapped Children Act of 1975, which provided the impetus for mainstreaming.

Subtly, the language describing the emphasis of schooling for students with developmental disabilities appeared to have shifted from 'train' to 'educate' in the 1970s. Not that the teaching of reading, writing and so on was totally ignored under the training or 'trainable' rubric, but the new educational zeitgeist had, it appeared, shifted to a more optimistic plane, one in which no student would be excluded from a programme of public education, one in which schooling would occur with nondisabled students to the maximum extent possible. Indeed, the new atmosphere held out the possibility that a person with Down syndrome could live a fulfiling adult life in the community if provided with an appropriate public school education in the least restrictive environmental possible, along with adequate educational supports while in school and beyond.

Against this background of events occurring in the 1960s and 1970s, an era still largely characterised by trainable placements, self-contained education and school eligibility uncertainty, the 171 students with Down syndrome represented in this research synthesis were entering schools or were in their early years of schooling.

The Minnesota/Illinois Studies

Over the last 30 years, three teams of researchers (Rynders and Horrobin; Abery; and Smith, Spiker, Peterson, Cicchetti and Justine) have gathered extensive cross-sectional and/or longitudinal psychoeducational measures describing the characteristics of 171 individuals with Down syndrome. Until now, however, many of the findings in these studies have not been combined so as to create an articulated set of findings that are both cross-sectionally and longitudinally interrelated. But, because the three directors or co-directors within the studies (Rynders, Abery, Spiker) planned in advance eventually to mesh their three sets of findings, it is now possible to describe the psychoeducational ability of individuals in their three cohorts. Both longitudinal and cross-sectional, this amalgamated data set reveals extensive information on the educational progress of a relatively large group of home-reared public school students with Down syndrome.

Let us look briefly at the basic details of the three studies from which the data-set amalgamation was created. Spiker and her associates (Smith et al. 1984) evaluated the effects of administering megavitamins and minerals on the intelligence of 56 school-aged children with Down syndrome living at home in the Chicago, Illinois area. Spiker's subjects were all karyotyped and 90 per cent had the regular trisomy 21 form of the syndrome (four of them had the translocation form; one had the mosaic form). Spiker's cohort expands the range of racial and educational diversity when combined with the other two studies; families in her cohort were more racially diverse than in either of the other studies, and the education level of parents ranged from less than high-school graduation (10%), to 39 per cent having no education beyond high school graduation, and 17 per cent who were college graduates. In her study, a two-group double blind clinical trial experiment was designed specifically to assess the efficacy of a megavitamin-mineral supplement, a supplement that had been proposed to be beneficial in terms of improving cognitive functioning in children with mental retardation (Harrell et al. 1981). Children of various ages with Down syndrome were evaluated individually at baseline, at four months, and again at eight months thereafter. Results revealed that the two matched groups were not significantly different in IQ, motor, language and other relevant test scores at either the four- or eight-month test periods, with the placebo group performing as well as the group receiving vitamin and mineral supplements on all criterion measures.

Abery (1988) employed a multi-method, multi-measure research design to investigate possible differences between the interaction styles of 63 families with children with Down syndrome and a matched sample of families with children of average intelligence on a cross-sectional basis. Children in Abery's study all had Down syndrome, based on physicians' findings as summarized by parents, with all but 12 of the parents being able to confirm that the karyotype was regular trisomy 21. Thus it is possible that a small number of children in his sample had either the mosaic or translocation form of the syndrome, though on a probabilistic basis the odds of that are relatively small. Nearly all of his families were Caucasian, and several parents had some years of higher education and above average incomes. Measures of family interaction were based on a number of self-report inventories and direct behavioural observation, and children's competence was based upon teacher ratings of classroom behaviour and a standardized measure of academic achievement. Families containing children with Down syndrome displayed a distinct, though functional, style of interaction that could be characterized as flexibly connected. Moderate levels of cohesion, the use of positive behavioural change strategies, and positive responsiveness from mothers, along with a number of other family variables, all correlated positively and significantly with teacher ratings of child competence within the classroom environment.

In 1968, Rynders, and his associate Horrobin, began a longitudinal early intervention study in the Twin Cities area called project EDGE (Expanding Developmental Growth through Education), beginning when the children with Down syndrome were infants. The sample contained 35 children (23 males and 12 females) all of whom had the regular trisomy 21 (nondisjunction) form of the condition as confirmed with karyotype records. Within the set of 35 families, the education level of the mothers and fathers averaged slightly above the high school graduation level and nearly all were Caucasian. Activities revolved around providing daily sessions of language-enriched play activities presented by children's parents (usually mothers). The infant-toddler phase was followed by a preschool programme where the language emphasis was maintained by early education teachers through a wide variety of activities. A distal control group living in Illinois, while involved in early intervention of various kinds, did not receive the EDGE curriculum. Baseline testing when children were 12 months old indicated that the two groups were not significantly different in terms of relevant family characteristics and child abilities. At the age of five years, however, while the experimental group of children was significantly advanced in the areas of intelligence and gross motor performance (when adjusted for gender proportion differences across the two groups), it was not significantly advanced in either recep-tive or expressive language, the criterion variables. Therefore, the authors concluded that their findings provided support for the early education movement in general, but not for the EDGE curriculum (Rynders and Horrobin 1980). Hence the curriculum has never been published.

In sum, the two studies involving Spiker and Abery were *not* education inter-vention studies. And Rynders' study, while producing educationally significant differences in some precriterion early education variables, did *not* produce significant differences in the criterion area. Thus, collectively, outcomes represented in the three studies should not be regarded as emanating from 'schooling hybridized' or 'hand-picked' groups of children. Rather the findings reported in this article represent, in my view, represent relatively conservative estimates of the abilities of the population of children with Down syndrome. However, as the amalgamation of findings is not seamless and the composite sample is not representative of the full gamut of racial, ethnic, socioeconomic and other population factors, generalization is limited.

For analysis purposes, assessment components collected across the three studies were knit together. The longitudinal[2] data set (Rynders) contains information from ages 6 to 18+ years on the same group of children (EDGE project, described earlier). The cross-sectional data sets (Abery and Spiker) incorporate contributions of data for age-matched subgroups of the children with Down syndrome at four age points: 7-9.9 years, 10-13.9 years, 14-17.9 years, and 18+ years (note that the age point 10-13.9 years was extracted from the longitudinal EDGE data set and included in the cross-sectional data set for continuity purposes). Accordingly, then, in combining the three separate data sets into the superordinate data set, children were grouped on the bases of age and type of assessment and were no longer treated as subjects from three separate studies except where longitudinal measures could not be combined logically with cross-sectional measures.

Results[3]

Let us look to IQ test results first. Examination of Table 6.1 reveals that IQ means decline as age progresses in both the longitudinal and cross-sectional samples. This is reflected in the evident trend shown within the table for percentages of children in higher intellectual categories to diminish over time. For example, in the cross-sectional data set, at the 7.0-9.9 age point 3.7 per cent have IQs in the borderline normal category, with 14 per cent in the severe mental retardation or below level. At age 18+, no individual is represented in the borderline normal category and 38.5 per cent fall in the severe mental retardation or below level. Note particularly, though, that there are large *individual* differences, as represented in the IQ score ranges and standard deviations at every age level.[4]

---

[2] Throughout the remainder of this paper wherever the word 'longitudinal' is used, it refers to individuals in the EDGE project data set.

[3] Tables and figures are reprinted, with permission, from the Rynders et. al. article in the Down Syndrome Quarterly, March 1997, Vol. 2, No. 1.

[4] It is important to note that in the cross-sectional portions of the tables to follow, and the analyses based on them, 12 persons in Abery's Study were not identifiable in terms of their Karyotypic Subtype of Down syndrome. Similary, in the Smith et al. Study, 5 individuals with confirmed Down syndrome, while known to have the translocation or mosaic subtype (N=4 and 1 respectively), are not identifiable as indvidual. Thus, the influence of low incidence Subtype and its affect on variance contribution, if present, is unknown. This is not the case in the longitudinal study where all individuals have regular trisomy 21.

Table 6.1 IQ scores* during the schooling period for individuals who have Down syndrome

IQ scores (full scale) (longitudinal) (Rynders, Horrobin)	Age				
Statistical measurement parameters	6.0–6.9	7.0–9.9	10.0–13.9	14.0–17.9	18+
Mean (M)	50.3	N/A	45.1	54.8	46.8
Standard deviation (SD)	11.9	N/A	9.9	7.5	9.8
Range	33–85	N/A	35–73	50–70	39–63
(N)	33	N/A	15	6	5
IQ percentage distribution (longitudinal)	Age				
Level of mental retardation	6.0–6.9	7.0–9.9	10.0–13.9	14.0–17.9	18+
% Low normal	3	N/A	0	0	0
% Borderline normal	3	N/A	6.7	16.7	0
% Mild mental retardation	30.3	N/A	0	0	20
% Moderate mental retardation	51.5	N/A	66.7	83.3	60
% Severe mental retardation or below	12.1	N/A	26.7	0	20
IQ scores (full scale) (cross-sectional) (Abery, Smith, Spiker, Peterson et al.: data sets combined)	Age				
Statistical measurement parameters	6.0–6.9	7.0–9.9	10.0–13.9	14.0–17.9	18+
Mean (M)	N/A	49.9	48.1	45	47.5
Standard deviation (SD)	N/A	12	10.4	7.7	12.4
Range	N/A	27–74	24–77	24–62	30–63
(N)	N/A	27	34	21	13
IQ Percentage distributions (cross-sectional)	Age				
Level of mental retardation	6.0–6.9	7.0–9.9	10.0–13.9	14.0–17.9	18+
% Low normal	N/A	0	0	0	0
% Borderline normal	N/A	3.7	8.8	0	0
% Mild mental retardation	N/A	29.6	8.8	9.5	30.8
% Moderate mental retardation	N/A	51.9	73.5	76.2	30.8
% Severe mental retardation or below	N/A	14.8	8.8	14.3	38.5

* Stanford-Binet norms, both traditional and 1982 versions, produced identical results except for the 6.0-6.9 age point, where the 1972 norm values were slightly lower (mean=47.2, SD=10.7, range=29-71) than the traditional norms.

In the longitudinal data set the cross-sectional data trend is repeated, with IQ means tending to drop over time and percentages of children and youth found within higher intellectual categories diminishing as well. It should be noted, however, that the number of individuals in the longitudinal set is modest (except for the 6.0-6.9 age point) due to the fact that the distal control group in the EDGE project was no longer in the follow-up portion of the study after the 6.0-6.9 age point since the federally funded early intervention programme ended at the age of 7.0 years.

Moving from IQ test results to language and motor outcomes (see Table 6.2), language and motor abilities are roughly equivalent to one-half of CA in terms of age equivalent scores at the 7.0-9.9 age point. Note, though, that students' progress, while modest, is moving upward across the schooling years. Indeed, progress across age in terms of the Peabody Picture Vocabulary Test (PPVT, Dunn and Dunn 1981) results is quite positive: an ANOVA (PPVT x CA) reveals a significant positive difference ($F=9.40$, $P<.01$) between PPVT scores across age points, but differences are not significant for the PPVT x gender analysis. Similarly, motor performance, measured on the Bruininks-Oseretsky test of motor proficiency (B-O, Bruininks 1978), shows positive growth across age, revealing a significant difference ($F=.89$, $P<.01$) for age but not for gender.

With regard to academic achievement, performance grows consistently across age points (see Table 6.3), but in relatively small increments.

In this table findings are displayed in terms of grade equivalents, not age equivalents, because I believe that teachers, school psychologists and other education personnel will appreciate them more fully in that form. The following grade equivalency scores from the Peabody Individual Achievement Test (PIAT, Dunn and Markwardt 1970) reveal significant positive change across age with all ages combined: reading comprehension ($F=4.34$, $P<.02$), reading recognition ($F=4.24$, $P<.02$), and spelling ($F=4.06$, $P<.02$). PIAT math grade equivalency scores were not significantly

Table 6.2 Language and motor scores of school-age students with Down syndrome (age equivalents)

Type of test		Age			
		7.0–9.9 (cross-sectional)	10.0–13.9 (cross-sectional)	10.0–13.9 (longitudinal)	14.0–17.9 (cross-sectional)
PPVT	M	3.7	4.9	5.4	5.9
	SD	0.99	1.3	1.2	1.7
	Range	2.1–5.6	2.3–8.5	3.3–7.1	3.7–9.0
	N	15	26	15	15
B-O	M	4.2	4.3	4.5	4.6
	SD	0.09	0.16	0.3	0.21
	Range	4.2–4.4	4.2–4.8	4.2–5.2	4.2–4.8
	N	12	24	15	16

Table 6.3 Academic achievement of school-age students who have Down syndrome (grade equivalents)

(Longitudinal) Type of test (PIAT)		Age			
		7.0–9.9	10.0–13.9	14.0–13.9	18+
Mathematics	M	N/A	0.83	1.7	1.7
	SD	N/A	0.86	0.83	1.1
	Range	N/A	0.1–2.7	0.5–2.5	0.1–4.9
	N	N/A	15	9	15
Reading recognition	M	N/A	3.3	3.6	4.2
	SD	N/A	2.1	1.8	2.4
	Range	N/A	0.8–8.9	1.5–6.0	0.9–9.6
	N	N/A	15	9	15
Reading comprehension	M	N/A	2.3	2.8	3.01
	SD	N/A	1.1	0.87	2.2
	Range	N/A	0.1–4.2	1.5–4.0	0.1–6.8
	N	N/A	15	9	15
Spelling	M	N/A	2.3	2.8	3.6
	SD	N/A	1.1	1.2	2.4
	Range	N/A	0.7–4.1	1.0–4.0	1.4–8.0
	N	N/A	15	9	15

(Cross-sectional) Type of test (PIAT)		Age			
		7.0–9.9	10.0–13.9	14.0–13.9	18+
Mathematics	M	0.63	0.86	1.1	1.4
	SD	0.39	0.58	0.68	0.58
	Range	0.1–1.5	0.5–2.0	0.5–2.0	0.5–2.0
	N	13	10	15	8
Reading recognition	M	1.2	2.01	3.01	3.9
	SD	0.62	1.2	2.3	2.01
	Range	0.1–2.5	0.5–4.0	0.5–7.0	1.5–7.5
	N	13	10	15	8
Reading comprehension	M	1.3	1.9	2.4	2.9
	SD	0.89	0.85	1.1	1.6
	Range	0.1–2.5	0.5–3.0	0.5–4.5	1.5–6.5
	N	13	10	15	8
Spelling	M	1.1	1.7	2.5	4.1
	SD	0.52	1.1	2	2.4
	Range	0.1–2.0	0.5–4.0	0.5–7.5	1.5–8.5
	N	13	10	15	8

different. With respect to PIAT grade equivalency scores by gender, reading comprehension ($F=4.30$, $P<.04$), and reading recognition ($F=5.07$, $P<.03$), were statistically significant, both of which favoured females. Other PIAT x gender differences were not significant statistically.

Of particular importance, at least in my view, is the row titled in both the longitudinal and cross-sectional sets as 'Reading comprehension'. PIAT reading comprehension items require individuals to read sentences, not just isolated words, and to extract their meaning. Achieving reading comprehension grade equivalent scores of 2.9 (cross-sectional) and 3.0 (longitudinal) by the age of 18+ years is indicative of reading ability that represents a level of literacy suitable for purposes such as reading a good share of the TV guide as well as portions of the newspaper, restaurant menus, and so on. In addition, several of the young adults read library books for their leisure enjoyment. This level of literacy attainment certainly exceeds the often prescribed target of teaching only a 'list of sight words for safety' expectation.

How do our findings in this portion of the paper square with other findings? Seeing IQ decline over an extended age span for individuals with Down syndrome who are well into their schooling years is not a surprise. Carr (1994) also noted this decline with age in an extensive review of the literature; but evidence just emerging suggests that this decline may, in some cases, not only be interrupted in adulthood but reversed (Carr 1994). Identifying the specific circumstances under which this reversal may occur will be an exciting topic for future research.

With respect to motor findings, delays in performance across the 171 individuals are consistent with Block's (1991) review in which he points out that motor delays are common in students with Down syndrome not only because of motor performance differences and challenges, but because of the physiological, medical and health characteristics associated with the condition.

Regarding receptive and expressive language and academics, this symbol acquisition and usage domain presents special challenges for most individuals who have Down syndrome, especially as symbol complexity increases (Cicchetti and Beeghly 1990).

As we shall see in the next section, a variety of educational approaches are showing particular promise in enhancing the learning of students who have Down syndrome in the areas of academics, motor and language.

Educational Implications

1. The designators 'trainable' and 'educable' are out of date and can be barriers to providing an appropriate education to students who have Down syndrome

As indicated near the beginning of this article, the terms, 'trainable' and 'educable' (IQ-linked designators up to the mid-1970s) exerted a powerful influence on the types of instructional activities and classroom placements that students with Down syndrome received, although the assessment of adaptive behaviour has given more balance to the process. IQ has been, and continues to be, correlated positively with certain indicators of school achievement, especially those indicators that are related closely to domains of the intelligence test itself. But evidently, school personnel consider factors beyond IQ in making pragmatic educational decisions. Indeed, in some instances, education assessment team members seem to virtually ignore the IQ boundaries that define 'educable' and 'trainable'. For example, Abery (1988), in one of the three data sets in the present research synthesis, collected standardized IQ scores on the 63 students in his study. He discovered that 48 per cent of those students, all of whom attended public schools in Minneapolis or St Paul, had IQs in the mild range of mental retardation, making them eligible for an 'educable' class, at least on the basis of an intelligence test. But the majority of them were in 'trainable' classes. Why? My guess is that many teachers continue to believe, unequivocally, that students with Down syndrome are 'always trainable'. Most assuredly they are *not* all trainable (see Tables 6.1-6.3 again). In effect, the term 'trainable' can create an artificial ceiling on educational opportunity for students who have Down syndrome and, thus, should be eliminated. And 'educable', while less limiting from an academic perspective, should also be eliminated because it has such a long tradition of self-containment. In their place I recommend the substitution of the general designator 'student with Down syndrome', with placement determination following functional assessment on a continuing basis.

2. Parents need to avoid the 'IQ trap' when advocating for an academically oriented school programme

Parents of children with Down syndrome need to be alerted to a problem or trap that they sometimes unwittingly create for themselves to step into. The 'trap' is actually a trapping misperception and is usually approached through a sequence of two steps, both of which involve an over-emphasis on IQ score:

Step 1. Because young children with Down syndrome often score in the mild mental retardation IQ range or above (see Table 6.1), parents may stress IQ level in making their initial argument for an academically oriented programme. Let us suppose that they are successful in their early efforts. So far, so good, but the trap is about to be sprung.

Step 2. Parents, having argued successfully for an academically oriented class placement based on an IQ in the mild range, continue to fight for a succession of similar class placements as their child grows older, basing their advocacy efforts on annual intelligence testing results. They now have all of their 'eggs in the IQ basket'. The trap is about to catch them though, because *the IQ scores of most children with Down syndrome will usually diminish as they grow older, making their parents' argument for an academically oriented placement increasingly difficult each year.*

It should not be surprising that IQ scores generally decrease with advancing age across individuals with Down syndrome, considering that they exhibit protracted rates of learning from a developmental perspective (Cicchetti and Beeghley 1990), and that their domain-specific learning profiles are not uniform across age (Cunningham 1988). Couple these factors with their special problems in complex verbal learning tasks (Rynders et al. 1979), task types which are featured heavily in IQ tests, and it would be surprising if the IQ scores of individuals who have Down syndrome did not decrease with increasing age. (Space limitations do not permit a full discussion of this complex topic. But the book by Rondal (1995), along with other sections of this book, will be very helpful in furthering the understanding of the relation between cognitive and language and other markers of symbol-related learning in persons who have Down syndrome.)

Frustration with educators' misunderstanding (and occasional misuse) of assessment data has led some parents and professionals to call for the abandonment of standardized intelligence testing altogether. I do not favour the abolition of intelligence testing because it provides a useful norm-referenced measure of general cognitive ability. However, parents of children with Down syndrome should insist that abilities central to the *substance* of **educateability** receive much more attention during the assessment and placement planning process. For example, during a placement conference, parents, if interested in promoting academic opportunities, should be encouraged to talk in detail about their child's interest in books, conceptualization ability, language repertoire, and quality of instructional socialization. These are important predictors of academic learning ability, with educational value far in excess of an IQ score by itself.

3. Teachers should expect to see positive and fairly continuous progress in achievement across the schooling years and will want to build upon it

Teachers' observations of the fact that IQ often diminishes as a child with Down syndrome matures may lead them to believe that achievement in motor, language and academics will decrease as well. But, as the results shown in Tables 6.2 and 6.3 reveal, students' achievement levels in receptive language, reading, fine and gross motor performance, and so on are generally improving. Indeed, PPVT, B-O, and the majority of PIAT scores are generally increasing, often significantly, across age. Moreover, increases are continuing into the secondary years and on into the young adult years as well. Thus, teachers' efforts to promote the capabilities of students with Down syndrome, if persistent and continuous, will usually be rewarded over the long term (again, see Tables 6.2 and 6.3). However, this does *not* mean that an 'academics at all costs' approach or something similar should be assumed. There is, after all, 'life after schooling,' and an individual with Down syndrome needs to learn how to do a job well, exhibit good manners, and so on, in addition to learning academic skills to a reasonable level of functional proficiency.

4. Teachers should assume a holistic approach to educating the child

Results shown in Tables 6.2 and 6.3 reveal that academic, motor and language capabilities are all generally increasing across age, though not all at the same rate or level. This suggests that these capabilities might be combined judiciously in learning opportunity provision so as to promote one another in a synergistic manner. This idea may not seem far-fetched when one considers that social and cognitive development have already been empirically demonstrated to be interrelated in children with Down syndrome (Cicchetti and Sroufe 1986).

Other forms of combination appear promising in the area of symbol learning, an area that is one of particular challenge for students with Down syndrome (see Nadel and Rosenthal 1995). For instance, combining manual with verbal communication activity, Miller et al. (1995) reported that children with Down syndrome can, with proper instruction, acquire a sign vocabulary which expands both their oral and signed vocabularies. Such instruction did not, by the way, inhibit children's development of oral language in any way. In a related vein, Oelwein (1995) took a game-like approach (eg, lotto) to helping students with Down syndrome organize symbolic information for memory filing, with promising early results.

Taking a multifaceted approach to speech and language improvement, Kumin et al. (1996) employed play activities to successfully facilitate higher-order play skills, and used computers to enhance language. In a similar vein, Meyers (1994) has demonstrated that with the use of computers, children with Down syndrome can be helped to bypass the pressing problems that often make speech signals and written texts inaccessible to them. For instance, in one of her studies she helped teenagers with Down syndrome learn to speak in sentences by having them work on computers with speech output capability. When writing a 30-page book (with assistance as needed), students used more than three times as many spontaneous grammatical sentences after ten sessions of computer writing as compared with a baseline period.

Finally, Buckley (1987) and Fowler et al. (1995) point to the advantages of teaching reading, language and writing together, showing that a dimension of language called phonological awareness (the ability to actively attend to the sound structure of language without regard to reading) was an area of weakness in participants with Down syndrome across all three types of activities.

Not that all activities should be conducted in this interrelated way, but some might lend themselves naturally and easily to an interrelated approach; and if the combinations are not 'forced' there may be, at the very least, additional interest value for some students in such activities.

Summary and Concluding Thoughts

Most of the 171 individuals with Down syndrome from the Minnesota/Illinois studies matriculated through programmes that were frequently segregated, not inclusionary, and many of these programmes were labelled as 'trainable'. Indeed, nearly all of the individuals in the three data cohorts were born, entering school, or in their early years of schooling in the 1960s and early 70s - long before US laws such as PL 94-142 guaranteed them a free public education in the least restrictive environment; before US laws such as PL 99-457 extended education down into the preschool and even the infancy period of life; and before the existence of most of the parent advocacy groups focused on Down syndrome. Yet, in spite of the absence of today's emphasis on inclusionary educational provisions, laws guaranteeing a free public education, and effective advocacy organizations, the children in the Minnesota/Illinois studies did remarkably well in terms of their educational achievements. Indeed, many of the 171 students across the three data cohorts achieved impressive levels of academic achievement in spite of the fact that the vast majority of their IQs were in the *moderate-not mild, not borderline*-level of mental retardation (see Table 6.1) throughout their prime years of schooling. Considering what these 171 students have achieved and the educational advances made since they were in public schooling back in the 1970s and 1980s, there is certainly every reason to be extremely optimistic about the educational future for individuals who have Down syndrome.

References

Abery B (1988) Family-Interaction and the School-Based Competence of Children with Down Syndrome. Unpublished doctoral dissertation, University of Minnesota.

Block M (1991) Motor development in children with Down syndrome: a review of the literature. Adapted Physical Activity Quarterly 8: 179-209.

Bruininks R (1978) Bruininks-Oseretsky Test of Motor Proficiency. Circle Pines, MN: American Guidance Service.

Buckley S (1987) Attaining basic educational skills: reading, writing, and numbers. In Lane D, Stratford B (eds) Current approaches to Down's syndrome. London: Holt, Rinehart and Winston. pp. 315-43.

Carr J (1994) Annotation: long-term outcome for people with Down syndrome. Journal of Child Psychology and Psychiatry 35, 3: 425-39.

Cicchetti D, Beeghly M (1990) Children with Down Syndrome: A Developmental Perspective. New York: Cambridge University.

Cicchetti D, Sroufe LA (1986) The relationship between affective and cognitive development in Down's syndrome infants. Child Development 47: 920-9.

Cruickshank W (1958) [Debate with Ignacy Goldberg.] The trainable but noneducable: whose responsibility. Journal of the National Education Association 47: 622-3.

Cunningham C (1988) Down's Syndrome: An Introduction for Parents. Cambridge, MA: Brookline Books.

Down JLH (1866) Observations on an ethnic classification of idiots. London Hospital, Clinical Lectures and Reports 3: 259-62.

Dunn L, Dunn L (1981) Peabody Picture Vocabulary Test. Circle Pines, MN: American Guidance Service.

Dunn L, Markwardt F (1970) Peabody Individual Achievement Test. Circle Pines, MN: American Guidance Service.

Ferguson P (1995) Introductory comments on Down's observations. Mental Retardation 33: 54.

Fowler A, Doherty B, Boynton L (1995) Basis of reading skills in young adults with Down syndrome. In Nadel L, Rosenthal D (eds) Down Syndrome: Living and learning in the Community. New York: Wiley-Liss. pp. 182-95.

Goldberg I (1958) [Debate with William Cruickshank.] The trainable but noneducable: whose responsibility. Journal of the National Education Association 47: 622-3.

Harrell H, Capp R, Davis D, Peerless J, Ravitz L (1981) Can nutritional supplements help mentally retarded children? An exploratory study. Proceedings: National Academy of Science, USA 78: 574-8.

Kumin L, Councill C, Goodman M (1996) Comprehensive speech and language intervention for school-aged children with Down syndrome. Down Syndrome Quarterly 1: 1-7.

Meyers L (1994) Teach me my language: using technology to teach spoken and written language. Proceedings, National Down Syndrome Congress 22nd Annual Convention, August 26-28.

Miller J, Leddy M, Julianna M, Sedey A (1995) The development of early language skills in children with Down syndrome. In Nadel L, Rosenthal D (eds) Down Syndrome: Living and Learning in the Community. New York: Wiley-Liss. pp. 115-20.

Nadel L, Rosenthal D (1995) Down Syndrome: Living and Learning in the Community. New York: Wiley-Liss.

Oelwein P (1995) Teaching Reading to Children with Down Syndrome: A Guide for Parents and Teachers. Bethesda, MD: Woodbine House.

Pennsylvania Association for Retarded Children vs. Commonwealth of Pennsylvania (1972). E.D.Pa.

Rondal J (1995) Exceptional Language Development in Down Syndrome. New York: Cambridge University Press.

Rynders J (1995) Supporting the educational development and progress of persons with Down syndrome. In Barclay A(ed) Caring for Individuals with Down Syndrome and their Families. The Third Ross Roundtable on Critical Issues in Family Medicine. Columbus: Ross Products Division, Abbott Laboratories.

Rynders J, Horrobin J (1980). Educational provisions for young children with Down's syndrome. In Gottlieb J (ed), Educating Mentally Retarded Persons in the Mainstream. Baltimore, MD: University Park Press. pp. 109-47.

Rynders J, Horrobin J (1990) Always trainable? Never educable? Updating educational expectations concerning children with Down syndrome. American Journal on Mental Retardation 95 1: 77-83.

Rynders J, Abery B, Spiker D, Olive M, Sheran C, Zajac R (1997) Improving educational programming for individuals with Down syndrome: engaging the fuller competence. Down Syndrome Quarterly 2, 1: 1-11.

Rynders J, Behlen K, Horrobin M (1979) Performance characteristics of preschool Down's syndrome children receiving augmented or repetitive verbal instruction. American Journal of Mental Deficiency 84, 1: 67-73.

Rynders J, Spiker D, Horrobin J (1978) Underestimating the educability of Down's syndrome children: examination of methodological problems in recent literature. American Journal of Mental Deficiency 82: 440-8.

Smith G, Spiker D, Peterson C, Cicchetti D, Justine P (1984) Use of megadoses of vitamins with minerals in Down syndrome. The Journal of Pediatrics 105, 2: 228-34.

Chapter 7
Inclusion: A Committed Form of Working in School

CARMEN GARCÍA PASTOR

Introduction

The purpose of this chapter is to explain inclusion as a committed way of working in school. To accomplish this goal we are going to view the opposite term, 'exclusive', in relation to all that is considered as a higher level, or elitist, and so on. We start by noting, from our own experience, our wishes of having 'exclusive' things or belonging to 'elite' groups.

We have generally considered the term 'exclusive' positively, because we have not paid enough attention to its real meaning: exclusive is something that is not for everyone; it is only for certain people. While this may be a legitimate choice in the private area, it is not in the public area. Obviously, 'public' and 'exclusive' are opposed terms too, although this is not so obvious if we look at the many public institutions, including schools, which function exclusively.

The fact that, in the past, many children with special needs were referred to special services is an example of how schools have selected the best students, poorly serving the goal of social equality. Schools have used several mechanisms to select children, but the main way has been by considering their ability to adapt to the unique curriculum and pedagogy offered (Carrier 1986). For many students education has become an obstacle race in which only the best reach the end. But, we can ask, the end of what? What is the purpose of this race? In what kind of society will the winners and those that left this race live? These questions are linked with another that is included in a wider debate that relates to mass education: What kind of society do we want to create and how can educational systems serve to create this society?

Our educational systems incorporate contradictions which impede the ability of public schools to accept the commitment to inclusive education, because at the same time they encourage democratic and meritocratic practices.

Education, Social Justice and Equity

Today, social justice is considered a key factor in the current debate within special education reform; in fact, part of the criticism extended to the field is linked to this notion. Christensen and Dorn (1997) point out that although the notions of social justice and equity have always been implicit in this debate they have rarely been discussed openly. From their point of view, behind common ideas about these notions there are very different perspectives on their meaning. In this sense, they are contested more than shared concepts.

Christensen and Dorn have considered two main perspectives or philosophies: individualist and communitarian. The individualist philosophy is characterized by arguments from Rawls (1971) and Nozick (1995), for whom individual liberty is a requisite for social justice, understanding that it might necessitate a limitation of inequality, perhaps in a compensatory way. In the case of Nozick's position 'it would justify inequality of cognition, as well as wealth, as an unfortunate necessity for guaranteeing the freedom to compete' (Christensen and Dorn 1997, p. 184). In this way it would be possible to consider that individualistic perspectives have argued for equality of access to public education and special treatment for students with special needs - because they conceptualize disability as inherent to individuals - justifying segregated settings as a compensatory way to offer more resources for the less able students.

For communitarian philosophies, however, society is not just a collection of atomized individuals, but 'a compact of people who share a core set of beliefs about living, and social justice should recognize the existence of those shared beliefs' (Christensen and Dorn 1997, p. 184). For these authors, communitarian perspectives appear to have no clearly articulated principles of justice, but an adequate position could be represented by Etzione (1993) who understands that 'justice would be a balance between responsibility and right, and the job of communitarians is to act whenever the balance is disturbed' (Christensen and Dorn 1997, p. 184).

The concept of responsibility is opportune for us because it refers to a wider social context in which individual rights have to be developed, and it should be explained why, in the case of special education reform, its own role within a wider educational and social context has been forgotten. In this sense, as Christensen and Dorn have pointed out, the predominance of individualistic assumptions has operated in the past two decades, serving people with disability poorly.

We could summarize the limitations of individualistic philosophies in terms of two main issues. First, when these perspectives emphasize the individual right to special treatment they forget the ecological contingencies of social and environmental interventions; thus these environments will always be 'restrictive', consecrating the contradiction between the principles of democratic schools and their inability to meet the needs of all their students. Second, the defence of individual rights has been linked to a gradual evolution in which the public culture of professions has been characterized by pragmatism and technical rationality (Ranson 1993), in order to accommodate what Elliott (1993) calls the 'social market': individualistic values associated with the social market model of public service provision 'celebrate corporate self-interest at the expense of teamwork, strategic collaboration and community service' (Hyland 1996, p. 540). Special education, and integration, is developed within the schemes of technical rationality, that is, because 'the field of educational administration is grounded in the notion of scientific management, an extremely narrow view which presupposes that organizational change is a rational-technical process' (Srktic 1991, p. 161). Thus special education has been conceived as a rational system that confers instructional benefits on students designated as handicapped.

What makes inclusion difficult

For special education practices the individualist perspective has meant the necessity of defining educational difficulties with respect to student characteristics. This position suggests that it is the individual with disability who has the problem and the intervention aims to provide him or her with the appropriate skills to cope with it. This perspective, inherited from the biological and psychological model of deviance, has been very influential in this field, although it is increasingly contested as many researchers and educators have acknowledged its negative effects. There are strong arguments for and against the individualist perspective. Ainscow (1995), for instance, summarizes the following five reasons:

1. labelling effects;
2. framework to meet special needs;
3. limiting opportunities;
4. resource provision;
5. maintenance of status quo.

Following the same scheme we are going to review some interesting contributions that reinforce these reasons. Most of the criticism of moves to special education has been provoked by the necessity to classify and the consequent effects of a categorical system and labelling. In previous work (García Pastor 1995) we reviewed this criticism through contributions from Scott and Douglas (1972), Gallager (1976), Apple (1979), Algozzine and Mercer (1980), Ysseldyke and Algozzine (1982), Bogdan and Kugelmass (1984) and Bogdan (1986).

Scott and Douglas (1972) argued that when someone has the label of deviant, the feeling emerges in the community that they have to do something with him/her. The most significant aspect of this reaction is that all 'help' is directed to the 'deviant' person, assuming that the causes of deviance are within him/her.

Apple (1979) followed the same argument, translating it into the school context to explain how, when we pay attention to students' problems, we do not attend to school problems and to conditions which have provoked the necessity of these constructs (deviance, disability and so on). Labels are not neutral and tend to become permanent, therefore a person who has been labelled remains in the assigned category. This could explain the particular relationship between school and students labelled as disabled, with low achievement or with learning disabilities. According to Apple, although these constructs are used to provide an appropriate education, it is also true that students may be damaged by this definition as people needing special treatment.

Gallager's view (1976) on 'profane uses' of labelling has become a common quotation for many authors (cf. Rowitz and Gunn 1984; Ysseldyke and Algozzine 1982). He considered that labelling serves to tranquilize professionals; it allows them to gain diagnostic closure on diffi-cult cases, followed by different programmes of treatment. Labelling also focuses the problem on the individual more than on complex and ecolog-ical conditions which might need social reform.

Algozzine and Mercer (1980) indicated that the effects of labelling may be studied from two perspectives: the impact of the label on the percep-tions and behaviour of the student him/herself, and the impact of the label on the perceptions and behaviour of others who interact with the student. They consider that labels provide a convenient reference point from which to make predictions as to the future of labelled individuals, as well as represent key words with which a variety of characteristics may be associ-ated: 'It is when implied stereotypical characteristics and/or expectations are negative that labels become a problem' (pp. 295-6).

Ysseldyke and Algozzine (1982) analysed studies in which effects of the mentally retarded label were reported, and summarized them according to three stages of transmission:

Stage 1: transmission to target (teacher, parent, nurse, trainee, caretaker);
Stage 2: transmission to subject (labelled child);
Stage 3: production of effect. Targets respond with behaviour appropriate to expectancy.

For these authors, it seems safe to conclude that labels are expectancy-generating stimuli, resulting in differential expectancy effects. The negative effects of the label 'mentally retarded' were evident in half of the 22 reviewed studies, although these are not the only biasing factors that may have contributed to the effects (Ysseldyke and Algozzine 1982, pp. 115-21).

Bogdan (1986) pointed out that individuals employing definitions of disabilities often mistake consensus for truth: 'Their constructions of 'reality' are seen as reality, and the commonality of definition helps to confirm this truth' (p. 346). Bogdan considers that disability, as special education constructs it, is a particular frame of mind by which to organize the world, a way to look at individual differences.

Rist and Harrel (1982) described the process in which teachers' expectations of their students are based on their definition of the child's handicapping conditions. With time, the student's achievement and behaviour is going to conform more and more closely with the original expectation of teachers.

The framework to meet educational needs has been also definitive: education for special needs students has meant 'treatment' - as a consequence of a medical model - and its derivation towards a more technical intervention was consecrated by a prescriptive teaching model. It is characterized by a link between disability and teaching efficacy. This approach tries to identify strengths and weaknesses in the student and to design instructional programmes based on the diagnosis:

> The model is rooted in the philosophy that academic and behaviour difficulties result from deficits, dysfunctions, or disabilities in the pupil and that it is necessary to remediate or compensate for, these disorders before the pupils can be expected to profit to instruction. (Ysseldyke and Algozzine 1982, p. 167)

The predominant conception of learning has provided this possibility of diagnosis, in this sense reflecting the work of Gagne (1967) in *Learning and Individual Differences*. As Deno (1990) has pointed out, if we compare this book with Ackerman et al. (1989) 20 years later we observe the same psychological approach. For Davidson (1988), methods of teaching pupils with special needs are increasingly becoming directly influenced by psychology, mainly by behavioural rather than cognitive models: 'because it is possible to produce packaged teaching programmes using a structured behavioural approach, apparently to fulfil teachers' needs for coherent and sequential materials to intervene in practice' (p. 170). Indeed, to reinforce this practice, legislation has provided the way for those other than teachers to prescribe how the students should be taught. Iano considers that when the teachers 'do not question the legitimacy of the broad educational contexts, practices and purposes within which their students are assigned to them for special services, and when they accept the role of helper or remediator within the boundaries and conditions established by others, then special education teachers are accepting a primarily technical role' (Iano 1990, p. 463). This mode of problem articulation and formulation is wholly technical, and it is derived from a more general technical interpretation of regular education in which teachers are neither expected nor required to examine critically or assess larger educational contexts, purposes, or ends. The fundamental decisions are made outside the classroom and school situation.

Iano (1990) has also pointed out that, as technicians, teachers accept problems and tasks as they are defined by others: 'That is, it is usually some kind of professional team in a school that diagnoses, labels, and classifies pupils as handicapped and in need of special educational services and teaching' (p. 463). From a technical view, teachers should primarily be concerned with methods and strategies for getting students to learn the prescribed content and skills, committing themselves to playing a technical role.

One of the negative effects of a technical perspective is the decontextualization of students' programmes from a general school curriculum, because according to the previous theory of learning, it is necessary to break down curricular units into smaller, isolated subcomponents. That is so in the prescriptive teaching model for which specific processes and abilities exist, although, as Ysseldyke and Algozzine (1982) noted, 'there is little empirical support for this contention' (p. 173).

For Iano (1990) it should be obvious that teachers do not merely 'produce' learning in students, because learning is not a matter of seeing if students achieve prescribed outcomes, but involves the joint transformation of teacher and students: 'this means that an intimate connection must be made between teachers' programming and their students' understandings and purposes' (p. 464).

Indeed, from this technical perspective it is possible that students work in isolation for too long, without the intellectual prompts, support and help provided by working in a group (Ainscow 1995). It is possible too that when he or she works in isolation different things are learned, and his or her education would be incomplete without an opportunity to be introduced to issues that promote (for his or her peers) 'an understanding of the world, sensitivity to the human condition, and reasoning and thinking skills during school years' (Stainback and Stainback 1990, p. 14). Thus it is important to evaluate the opportunities the student is missing in order to have time for learning what is considered as 'adequate' for him or her in an individual programme.

The conception of two different kinds of programme to adapt teaching to individual characteristics generates the idea that to meet special needs resources must be provided (Ainscow 1995). When there are few resources inclusion seems impossible, and schools generally do not have enough resources because they always need to improve their conditions. But conditions depend on many factors, from ideological ones to the delivery of resources, in different countries: if we look at less developed countries we can understand that inclusion means different realities, as my colleague Naicker explains: 'the actual form inclusive education takes will depend on human resources, the state of development of the educational system related to education training, physical facilities, fiscal resources, the extent to which the concept has been debated and the value attached to human dignity...' (Naicker and García Pastor, in press). In

South Africa, for example, the estimated 40-50 per cent failure and attrition rate of the approximately ten million children in the country makes the continued existence of segregated provision look ridiculous.

On the other hand, if we look at developed countries - the USA for instance, in which special education has enjoyed unprecedented support for nearly three decades, in terms of fiscal, political, legislative and human resources (with funding increasing from $37 million to upwards of $1 billion, from 1967 to 1980) - the field is receiving serious criticism from within and outside: 'Such criticism specifically includes the degree to which special education has failed to provide different set of experiences tailored to the individual needs of students with mild handicaps, despite the labels students carry' (Pugach 1990, p. 329).

Lastly, the individualist perspective, focusing the problem on the child, prevents the school from recognizing its own problems and its own way of improvement, so maintaining the status quo (Ainscow 1995). A status quo in which 'dominant discourses in special education are ill-equipped to penetrate beyond procedural issues and consider more fundamental questions about the future nature of education for all children' (Vicent and Evans 1996: 475).

Towards a New Professional Commitment

According to Skrtic (1996), much like all professional knowledge, that of special education is based on the positivist theory, assuming the following hierarchy: basic knowledge, applied knowledge and professional knowledge. Thus, on this basis, a particular conceptualization has determined development and practices in special education. But when this basic knowledge is contested, what happens to professional practices? For Skrtic this crisis could liberate professionals from conventional thinking, permitting them to consider alternative perspectives on which their practices could be based.

Traditional knowledge has generated a particular 'culture' characterized by the particular ways in which professionals deal with problems, thinking and solving them. When basic knowledge is contested this implies deep changes for practice. Moreover, changes do not refer to the individual but to a collective change within a reflective discourse, which has to create a new system of relationships to encourage the necessary conditions. As we have pointed out before (García Pastor 1997), in the actual scheme of practice, specialists make diagnoses and prescribe treatments, support teachers are responsible for individual programmes and classroom teachers execute part of them (in the same sense as described by Iano (1990)). This scheme perpetuates the traditional practice supported by an organizational system that educational administration reinforces, reinforcing at the same time the implicit hierarchy of knowledge, in which each professional is placed in a determinate level: knowledge is not shared, it flows in a top-down way.

Conditions for change are linked to the elimination of these hierarchies in order to share new knowledge in new schemes for professional collaboration, through new ways of communication to invent and reinvent new solutions to solve educational problems in their context (ad hoc). In this sense, although school organization is an example of a bureaucratic machine, this configuration could be changed under the organizational contingencies of collaboration, mutual adjustment and discursive coupling (Srktic 1991), so that traditional culture is replaced by a community of interests.

Professional interests must focus on the promotion of collective life as opposed to individual interests, because the 'public dimension' of education implies that 'teachers have duties and concerns which transcend those of professionals in the private sector' (Bottery and Wright 1996, p. 88). For these authors it is implicit within the role of public professionals that they need to consider the nature of this role, but within a societal context as well. In this way, teachers and other professionals in schools need to revise their roles, referring to individual differences and the dominant perspective to meet them, because they have to consider a more balanced perspective of social justice and equity, recognizing diversity as a human condition and individual rights to an adequate education within a wider concept of social responsibility, of communality. This is necessary because teachers and other school professionals have to understand the political, social and ethical implications of their practices.

Change is not easy, because professional culture in special education, as in the culture of most public service professions, is characterized by pragmatism and technical rationality (Hyland 1996; Ranson 1993), as we have pointed out above. Efficiency has been the priority above other social goals, and professional studies, education and training are accommodated in this 'social market'. In this context, theoretical knowledge in training is a purely technical or instrumental one, operating as 'an ideological device for eliminating values issues from domains of professional practice' (Elliot 1993, p. 23).

These circumstances, together with recent policy developments in special education, have important effects on 'professionalism', based on the necessity for 'technical competence' to meet special needs. As Fulcher (1989) has pointed out, there are two main arguments against professionalism: it is 'anti-democratic, because it excludes the person most affected from taking the decision' (p. 24) and it is strategic - 'it is deployed as a retreat from responsibility (your child not mine)' (p. 24). Fulcher's criticism against professionalism implies a view of bureaucratic practices in which 'experts' have demarcated areas of responsibility: 'the notion of expertise increases the likelihood that professionalism is deployed' (p.24).

Nevertheless it is very important to change from this 'social market' model towards the new model of 'work-based learning' as it becomes possible to renew professional values and commitment in the public services. It is in this sense that inclusion means a committed way of working in school, because 'an inclusive school is a place where everyone belongs, is accepted, supports, and is supported by his or her peers and other members of school community in the course of having his or her educational needs met' (Stainback and Stainback 1990, p. 3).

Skrtic et al. (1996) suggest that inclusive education provides the place and the catalyst through which general education and special educators, students and parents can come together to create quality, democratic schools. For them, even the term inclusion has been used so widely that it has almost lost its meaning. The original sense can be defined in a few words: 'inclusive schools are those designed to meet educational needs of all their members within common environments and activities', as it was defined by Sapon-Shevin (1992, p. 20). This definition emphasizes the main idea that the 'inclusion movement represents school improvement on many levels for all students, not just the physical placement of individuals with various disabilities in general classrooms' (Skrtic et al. 1996, p. 149). For these authors inclusion can be seen as the latter of two phases of an 'equity movement': in the first phase, or integration, the equity movement did not question the structure of schools, but, in fact, the requirements for meeting special needs imply more and more changes in school organization, in such a way that each school becomes different because of the variety of needs and ways to meet them. Thus, the second phase was generated by the necessity of school restructuring, advocating a 'totally adaptive system of education'.

This explanation is based on the American context, yet it is true for others also. In the case of the United Kingdom, for instance, criticisms of the politics of 'special educational needs' developed after the 1981 Education Act advocated a 'whole-school approach', similar in most ways to the assumptions of the inclusion movement in the USA. In fact, the same concept of 'special needs education' was an important key, because to deal with the categorical system of identification and classification was the first step to advancing the restructuring of the system of education.

As Udvari-Solner and Thousand (1996) point out, inclusion is qualitatively different from integration or mainstreaming efforts of the past, which attempted to 'fit' a particular category of students. It is 'a process of operating in a classroom or school as a supportive community' which 'requires a curriculum and instructional practices that are responsive and inherently accommodating to nontraditional learners as well as those students with significant educational needs' (p. 182).

Many people do not take into account the fact that the whole is more than the sum of its parts, and when special and general education are unified a new system of education emerges: that is, a new conception of school that we now call inclusive, and which defines our challenge for the future. As Stainback and Stainback have stressed, the major reason for inclusion is not that previously excluded students are necessarily going to become proficient, although it is obvious that there are more opportunities for everyone in inclusive classrooms. 'Rather, inclusion of all students teaches the students and his or her peers that all persons are equally valued members of this society and that it is worthwhile to do whatever it takes to include everyone' (Stainback and Stainback 1990, p. 3). Maybe some people think that is a dream, but perhaps one which can come true depending on our professional commitment and collaborative work with students, parents and the whole community.

References

Ackerman P, Stenberg R, Glaser GR (eds) (1989) Learning and Individual Differences. New York: Freeman.

Ainscow M (1995) Necesidades Educativas Especiales. Madrid: Narcea.

Algozzine B, Mercer CD (1980) Labels and expectancies for handicapped children and young. In Mann L, Sabatino DA (eds) Four Reviews of Special Education. New York: Grune.

Apple MW (1979) Ideología y Curriculo. Madrid: Akal.

Barton L (1994) Teacher education and professionalism in England: some emerging issues. British Journal of Sociology of Education 15, 4: 529-43.

Bogdan R (1986) A sociology of special education. In Morris RJ, Blatt B (eds) Special Education: Research and Trends. Oxford: Pergamon Press. pp. 334-59.

Bogdan R, Kugelmass J (1984) Case studies of mainstreaming: a symbolic interactionist approach to special schooling. In Barton L, Tomlinson S (eds) Special Education and Social Interests. London: Croom Helm. pp. 173-91.

Bottery M, Wright N (1996). Cooperative in their deprofessionalitation? On the need to recognise the 'public' and 'ecological' roles of the teaching profession. British Journal of Educational Studies 44, 1: 82-98.

Carrier JC (1986) Sociology and special education: differentation and allocation in mass education. American Journal of Education, May, 281-93.

Christensen C, Dorn S (1997) Competing notions of social justice and contradictions in special education reform. The Journal of Special Education 31, 2: 181-98.

Davidson B (1988) The curriculum: some issues for debate. In Barton L (ed) The Politics of Special Educational Needs. London: The Falmer Press. pp. 161-74.

Deno S (1990) Educating students with mild disabilities in general education classroom: Minnesota alternatives. Exceptional Children 57, 2: 109-15.

Elliot J (1993) (ed) Reconstructing Teacher Education. London: Falmer Press.

Etzione A (1993) The Spirit of Community: Rights, Responsibilities, and the Communitarian Agenda. New York: Croom Helm.

Fulcher G (1989) Integrate and mainstream? Comparative issues in the politics of these policies. In Barton L (ed) The Integration: Myth or Reality. London: The Falmer Press. pp. 6-29.

Gagne RM (1967) Learning and Individual Differences. Columbus, OH: Merrill.

Gallager JJ (1976) The sacred and profane uses of labeling. Mental 3: 7.

García Pastor C (1995) Una Escuela Común para Niños Diferentes: La Integración Escolar (2ª edn). Barcelona: EUB.

García Pastor C (1997) La construcción de una escuela democrática. In Arnaiz P, De Haro P (eds) 10 Años de Integración en España: Análisis de la Realidad y Perspectivas de Futuro. Murcia: Publicaciones de la Universidad de Murcia.

Hyland T (1996) Professionalism, ethics and work-based learning. British Journal of Educational Studies 44, 2: 168-80.

Iano R (1990) Special education teachers: Technicians or educators. Journal of Learning Disabilities 23, 8: 462-5.

Naicker S, García Pastor C (in press) La reforma de la educación especial en Sudáfrica. Revista de Educación Especial.

Nozick R (1995) Anarchy, State and Utopia. New York: Basic Books.

Pugach M (1990) Commentary. The moral cost of retrenchment in special education. The Journal of Special Education 24, 3: 326-33.

Ranson S (1993) Markets or democracy for education. British Journal of Educational Studies 41, 4: 333-52.

Rawls J (1971) A Theory of Social Justice. Cambridge, MA: Belnap.

Rist R, Harrell J (1982) Labeling and the learning disabled child: the social ecology of educational practice. American Journal of Ortopsychiatry 52, 1: 146-60.

Rowitz L, Gunn E (1984) The labelling of educable mentally-retarded children. In Barton L, Tomlinson S (eds) Special Education and Social Interests. London: Croom Helm. pp. 149-72.

Sapon-Shevin T (1992) Celebrating diversity. In Stainback S, Stainback W(eds) Curriculum Considerations in Inclusive Classrooms: Facilitating Learning for all Children. Baltimore MD: Brooks.

Scott A, Douglas JD (1972) Theoretical Perspectives on Deviance. New York: Basic Books.

Srktic TM (1991) The special education paradox: equity as the way to excellence. Harvard Educational Review 61, 2: 148-206.

Srktic TM (1996) Crisis en el conocimiento de la educación especial: Una perspectiva sobre la perspectiva. In Franklin BM (ed) La Interpretación de la Discapacidad. Teoría e Histotia de la Educación Especial. Barcelona: Pomarés-Corredor.

Srktic TM, Sailor W, Gee K (1996) Voice collaboration and inclusion. RASE 17, 3: 142-7.

Stainback W, Stainback S (1984) A rationale for the merger of special and regular education. Exceptional Children 51, 2: 102-11.

Stainback W, Stainback S (1990) Support Networks for Inclusive Schooling. Baltimore, MD: Brookes.

Udvari-Solner A, Thousand JS (1996) Creating a responsive curriculum for inclusive schools. Remedial and Special Education 17, 3: 182-92.

Vicent C, Evans H (1996) Professionals under pressure: the adminsitration of special education in a changing context. British Educational Research Journal 22, 4: 475-91.

Ysseldyke JE, Algozzine B (1982) Critical Issues in Special and Remedial Education. Boston: Houghton Mifflin Company.

Chapter 8
Assistive Technology Compensating People with Down Syndrome

JAN-ERIK WÄNN, LARS-ÅKE BERGLUND AND ANDERS BOND

Assistive technology (AT) has the potential to be one of the main ways for people with Down syndrome to achieve both integration in society and an independent life.

When introducing AT into the lives of people with Down syndrome it is important to have a solid theoretical base and to make a thorough analysis of needs, possibilities and difficulties. There are two main reasons for this scientific approach. First, in a world with limited resources and limited funds it is imperative to find an economic solution by using technology appropriate to the situation. Secondly, AT, if wrongly adapted, might be a hindrance to independence. A person might become a slave to technology if he/she cannot master the assistive device.

Our analyses are based on the International Classification of Impairments, Disabilities, and Handicaps (ICIDH) which gives the following definition of handicap:

> In the context of health experience, a handicap is a disadvantage for a given individual, resulting from an impairment or a disability, that limits or prevents the fulfilment of a role that is normal (depending on age, sex, and social and cultural factors) for that individual. (WHO 1980, p. 183)

It also states that 'handicaps thus reflect interaction with and adaptation to the individual's surroundings' (WHO 1980, p. 14).

The Standard Rules on the Equalization of Opportunities for Persons with Disabilities (United Nations 1995) declares that:

> The term 'handicap' means the loss or limitation of opportunities to take part in the life of the community on an equal level with others. It describes the encounter between the person with a disability and the environment. The purpose of this term is to emphasize the focus on the shortcomings in the environment and in many organized activities in society, for example, information, communication and education, which prevent persons with disabilities from participating on equal terms. (United Nations 1995)

How can we focus on the shortcomings of the environment in an analysis? The following figures explain our method of thinking.

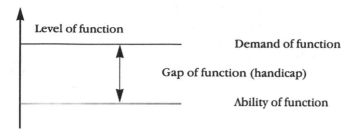

Figure 8.1 Level of function.
From: Borg et al. 1995, p. 19.

When the level of a function does not reach the level demanded by the environment there is a gap of function and the person has a handicap in that situation. It is important to remember in the analysis that a person has different functions, such as mobility, vision, hearing and cognitive. People with Down syndrome might have lower levels of ability than the situation demands for different functions, but here we are only going to talk about the cognitive function, as this usually is the main disability.

The level of each function and the situational demand for each function has to be assessed in order to find the 'problem' or 'bottleneck' in a given situation. Often there are just one or two minor bottlenecks in a complex situation. If we can find and compensate for these, we can eliminate the handicap. One example could be a person with Down syndrome who cannot prepare his/her own food. When analysing the situation we find that the problems are: a) the person cannot measure the ingredients correctly; and b) he/she does not know how to turn on the right plate on the stove. When we know the bottlenecks we can eliminate them by: a) using an electronic scale or ready made measures for that specific dish; and b) by painting the same colour on the turning knob and the plate it's regulating.

There are different ways of reducing the gap of function, as can be seen in Figure 8.2.

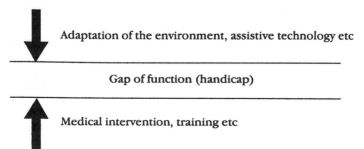

Figure 8.2 Reducing the gap of function.

The gap of function might be reduced by enhancing the level of function either through training, therapy or medical intervention. Every individual has an upper limit for how much the level of function might be enhanced and, of course, we should try to get the individual to reach that level. But it is also important to use the other way of reducing the situational demand mainly through adaptation of the environment and with technical aids. This is what we call assistive technology (Borg et al. 1995). People with cognitive disability (that might be caused by Down syndrome) usually have problems with short-term memory and level of abstraction. AT should reduce the demands on these two functions.

In our further analysis of the cognitive disability we use the theory developed by Kylen (Granlund et al. 1995) on cognitive functions in persons with mental retardation. The theory is based on theories by Guilford, Leeper, Thurstone and Piaget. In the theory there are four levels of abstraction. The first (the A-level) defines profound mental retardation; the second (the B-level) defines severe to moderate mental retardation; the third (the C-level) defines moderate to mild mental retardation. The fourth is the level for persons without mental retardation. The findings and devices presented in this article mainly concern adults at the B-level.

The Kylen theory further contains the following five cognitive content categories (Granlund et al. 1995):

- Quality, eg, how does the person classify common objects?
- Causal pattern, eg, how many links in a causal chain can the person understand?
- Space, eg, can the person find his/her way with the help of a map?
- Quantity, eg, how does the person handle money?
- Time, eg, can the person use a watch?

The assessment of needs for compensation, following the above mentioned theories, and a careful analysis of context and tasks is necessary before the AT is introduced. A useful sequence to follow is to find the bottlenecks and eliminate them by lowering the demand on the level of abstraction in concepts and operations.

The best technology is where the original designs are already made for 'all' persons. To avoid handicap in today's society, however, we often need special devices to compensate for the loss of cognitive function for people with Down syndrome. The following are two examples of assistive devices specially designed to compensate cognitive disabilities and to enhance independent living.

Time Aid

Our first example is a time aid, the quarter-hour watch (QHW) as described by Berglund and Bond (1995).

Time is an abstraction based on the perception of sequence and duration of events. We measure time with clocks and watches that indicate the momentary value in a theoretically defined time variable. Using a watch in a practical situation, for example to estimate the time remaining until a certain event, presupposes a series of abstract processes. You must know the time value of the anticipated event and subtract that value from the value shown by the watch. Furthermore, to make the result of this mathematical operation meaningful it must be related to previous experience of events or activities that could be contained within this framework.

The analysis above clearly shows why many persons with limited cognitive abilities do not find an ordinary watch useful and need a time aid to make it possible to handle the dimension of time. The QHW was developed in order to meet that demand.

The approach adopted was to design a watch that does not show the actual time, but gives a visual representation of the amount of time remaining until an event that the user chooses. This reduces the demand for abstract operations in a significant way and in a sense makes the dimension of time visible. It gives the user the opportunity to handle quantities of time in analogy with physical quantities.

In the area of making estimates of quantities, persons with developmental disabilities generally have pronounced problems in situations demanding response to changes in a dimension that has a continuous variation. For that reason the watch was given a time scale with discrete steps, each step representing a quarter of an hour. The choice of the 15-minute period as a unit gives a scale with relatively few steps, but still makes it possible to associate the duration of many common daily events with different values in the scale.

It is fully the responsibility of the user to activate the watch by choosing the event to relate to. Our experience is that people with developmental disabilities seldom have pronounced problems keeping track of the sequence of events in their life. The duration of events is the main problem.

To make a technical aid fit for use and attractive it is important that it is simple and offers the user the support he or she desires without unnecessary functions. It is important that the user experiences that the technical aid supports independence on his or her own terms; that it does not restrict freedom by having unnecessary elements of control or automation.

Alternative Keyboard

For people with cognitive disabilities the computer can be of immense help. However, the interface to the computer is seldom adapted to a person who cannot read or write but still wants to work independently. The following assistive device is designed primarily for people with cognitive disabilities, but people with mobility or visual problems will also benefit from its use.

The Flexiboard is an alternative keyboard, which a disabled person can independently use, with a great number of pictures, icons or other symbols to communicate with the computer. It is adaptable, with 128 programmable pressure sensitive surfaces that can be defined separately or grouped together. It has a built-in optical overlay detection, which means that different overlays are automatically recognized and exchange of overlays is done without commands to the computer.

The overlay definitions are stored in the Flexiboard, so that it can be moved from one computer to another maintaining the same function. The Flexiboard also gives adaptation possibilities for different kinds of motor disabilities, as the pressure sensitivity parameters can be set individually for each overlay.

It is possible for users to create their own overlays with a program that is included. The overlays, including both texts, pictures and optical coding, can be printed out on an ordinary printer.

Conclusions

The above-mentioned assistive devices were both developed after theoretical analysis of needs and assessments of bottlenecks. Both devices have been available for some years, mainly in the Scandinavian countries, and several hundred have been sold.

The introduction of a new technical aid to an individual with a developmental disability often generates special problems associated with difficulties in understanding instructions and the motivation to use the aid. According to our experience these problems can be minimized if technical aids for this group are designed to give the user an optimal chance to explore the product and gradually master the aid at his/her own pace. Persons with developmental disabilities are often confronted with various problems in their daily life and consequently they have experience as problem solvers. A well-designed technical aid can take advantage of this.

At the introduction of a QHW to a user the instructions are kept to a minimum, mainly focused on putting in and removing the coded picture card. Still, almost every one of the users gradually begins to utilize the information on the duration of time that the indicators on the watch provide.

Technical aids for people with cognitive disabilities need to incorporate the essential characteristic of contributing both to an enhanced quality of life for the user and providing the prerequisites for a more efficient use of socio-economic resources.

References

Berglund L-Å, Bond A (1995) The quarter hour watch, a time visualisation aid for persons with developmental disabilities. Proceedings of the Resna '95 Annual Conference. Vancouver: Resnapress. pp. 623-6.

Borg J, Turner-Smith A, Wänn J-E (1995) Assistive Technology - An Introduction. Stockholm: Handikappinstitutet.

Granlund M, Bond A, Lindström E, Wennberg B (1995). Assistive technology for cognitive disability. Technology and Disability 4: 204-14.

United Nations, Utrikesdepartementet, Socialdepartementet (1995) Standardregler för att tillförsäkra människor med funktionsnedsättningar delaktighet och jämlikhet. Stockholm: Gotab.

WHO (1980) International Classification of Impairments, Disabilities, and Handicaps. Geneva: WHO.

PART 4
PSYCHOLOGY, LANGUAGE AND COMMUNICATION

Chapter 9
Promoting the Cognitive Development of Children with Down Syndrome: The Practical Implications of Recent Psychological Research

SUE BUCKLEY

Introduction

Over the last 20 years there has been a considerable amount of research into the psychological development of children with Down syndrome, increasing our understanding of many aspects of their social, behavioural and cognitive development. It would not be possible to outline progress in all these areas in the space available. I have therefore chosen to focus on cognitive development as the area in which I have the greatest expertise and where I think that we are beginning to make considerable progress, with findings that lead us to be able to develop and evaluate practical interventions.

What is Cognitive Development?

Cognitive development may be described as the development of the mental abilities of talking, thinking, reasoning and remembering which underpin intelligence or intelligent behaviour. It is the slow development of these mental abilities that is probably the major concern of parents of children with Down syndrome, since they influence all aspects of understanding and controlling daily lives and determine the rate at which an infant can acquire knowledge about their world.

The Role of Speech and Language in Cognitive Development

I am going to argue that learning to talk has a central role in the development of mental abilities in a number of ways. Words equal knowledge, words are used for thinking, reasoning and remembering, and words support social communication and friendships.

Words for knowledge

Each word that a baby learns is an item of information about the world. As toddlers learn to talk the first words that they learn are for people, things and actions in their everyday world, labels for things that they see or experience. However, once children get started on this language pathway, we are able to talk to them about things that they are not experiencing. For example we can talk about what we did yesterday or what we are going to do tomorrow. We can talk about what doctors do in the hospital, about what happens in other countries and we can draw children's attention to new concepts and ideas through language. We have words for everything that we know something about, certainly if we are able to share that information with others. We add to our vocabularies throughout our lives and the size of our vocabularies will reflect the extent of our knowledge of the world. The speed at which a child is acquiring a vocabulary will influence the speed at which he or she is able to learn about the world that they live in.

Words for thinking, reasoning and remembering

Once a child begins to master language, first vocabulary and then grammar to build sentences, it becomes a very powerful tool. We use inner speech for thinking, reasoning, problem solving, remembering and organizing our behaviour. I am not suggesting that words are the only tools for mental representation, since we have visual imagery, smell imagery and so on, but I am arguing that language is by far the most powerful system for supporting learning and thinking, the core activities for mental development. It follows then, that any child with a significant delay in mastering language will be cognitively delayed and conversely, if we can improve their speech and language development we should improve their ability to think, reason, remember and learn.

Language and auditory short-term memory

Speech and language skills have also been shown to have a critical role to play in the development of auditory short-term memory in children. This is the system which holds incoming sensory information long enough for the brain to process it for meaning (not to be confused with long-term memory which is not generally impaired in persons with Down syndrome). The capacity of this auditory short-term memory system can be measured by finding out how many digits, said in random order at the rate of one per second, a child can repeat immediately in the same order. Typically, this span increases during childhood from about three digits at 4-5 years to six to seven digits at 16 years. Research has indicated that this system reflects the listener's efficiency at speech perception and speech production and children usually get quicker at recognizing and reproducing speech as they get older as a result of practice. Children's spans at any age, therefore, are approximately what they can say in two seconds. Research has shown that the efficiency of this auditory short-term memory system influences the speed at which children learn new vocabulary and learn to read. It is also thought to play a significant role in the processing and comprehension of speech and in organizing speech production (Gathercole and Baddeley 1993, Gathercole 1998). For children with Down syndrome this system is not usually increasing with age at a typical rate and most teenagers and adults only have spans of two to four digits (Buckley 1993, 1995a, b; Mackenzie and Hulme 1992).

Speech and language development in children with Down syndrome

There has been a great deal of research describing the speech and language development of children with Down syndrome over the past 20 years. Readers wishing to obtain more detailed information or read the evidence that supports the following summary are recommended to consult the reviews provided by Chapman 1995, 1997a, 1997b; Fowler 1995; Rondal 1995.

We now have consistent evidence to conclude the following for the majority of children with Down syndrome:

1. Speech and language abilities lag behind nonverbal reasoning abilities, so the children can be considered to have specific speech and language impairments (Chapman 1995, 1997b).
2. Speech production lags behind comprehension. For toddlers, first words are delayed relative to comprehension and then once the children get beyond two-word phrases, the ability to produce sentences lags behind sentence comprehension (Miller, 1988).
3. Vocabulary learning is ahead of grammar learning so teenagers will usually have vocabulary comprehension ages that are ahead of their grammar comprehension ages (Chapman 1997a).
4. Grammar is an area of particular difficulty and, while bound morphemes such as plural s, possessive s, and tense markers such as -ing and -ed are steadily mastered, the closed class grammar or function words are often still missing. These are articles (eg, a, the), verb auxiliaries (eg, is, are), pronouns (eg, she, her, I, them) and prepositions (eg, in, by, under). This slow and incomplete mastery of grammar results in rather 'telegraphic' speech, for example 'me sit chair' instead of 'I am going to sit on the chair' (Buckley 1993, 1995).
5. Speech intelligibility is usually poor. Most children have difficulty producing clear words and this is even harder for them when producing sentences (Stoel-Gammon 1997).

6. Most children with Down syndrome have good communication skills relative to their speech and language abilities. They are keen to be socially interactive and make good use of nonverbal skills such as eye-contact, smiling, turntaking and will often use natural gesture or sign to make themselves understood when their speech fails to get their message across.

7. There is great variability among children with Down syndrome in all aspects of development including speech and language development. Most children begin to use words between two and four years and slowly but steadily progress to be able to use intelligible sentences, albeit with limited grammar, by the time they are teenagers, adding to their vocabulary over time. However, some children have more profound speech and language impairments, make much slower progress and may rely on single words and signs to communicate as adults.

Some of the reasons for these difficulties

If we are going to try and improve the development of speech and language skills for the children we need to identify as many of the specific reasons for the above characteristics as possible. We have some pointers but by no means a complete picture of the causes let alone their interactive effects on the children's progress.

1. Hearing loss. There are consistent reports highlighting the high risk of mild to moderate hearing loss for children with Down syndrome. This is usually conductive loss due to glue in the middle ear and therefore fluctuating over time. There is also an increased likelihood of sensorineural loss and this will have a permanent effect on hearing ability. In my view, the significance of this high incidence of hearing loss on language learning is still underestimated. The long-term effects of glue ear are also not trivial. Marcell et al. have demonstrated that as many as 50 per cent of young adults may have permanent middle ear dysfunction and that these young people have poorer speech and language skills than those without the loss (Marcell 1995). Not only was their language knowledge less, they were also impaired on immediate speech recognition tasks.

2. Auditory discrimination. In our practical experience, we also see children who have difficulty in discriminating between similar sounding words, such as dolly and lolly, red and bread, horse and sauce, even when their hearing is within normal limits. This will make it very difficult to learn to understand the words that they are hearing as toddlers and slow up vocabulary comprehension considerably.

3. Auditory short-term memory. I have already drawn attention to the poor development of auditory short-term memory span for most children with Down syndrome and research on its significance in typically developing children indicates that this will also delay vocabu-

lary learning. It might be predicted to have an even bigger negative effect on the children's ability to master grammar as this will usually require the ability to hold a whole phrase or sentence in short-term store in order to process it for meaning.

4. Speech motor difficulties. The unclear speech of most children is likely to be due to a number of difficulties ranging from less effective operation of some or all of the brain mechanisms needed to plan and organize speech production to difficulties in moving the oral facial muscles and tongue with precision. Even if these speech mechanics work effectively, the children may be having difficulty in hearing speech sounds and word patterns clearly enough to establish good templates to guide their production.

Implications for effective interventions

Clearly there are a whole range of possible areas to target, starting with treating the hearing difficulties as effectively as possible to reduce their effects on both language and speech. In my view, activities aimed at encouraging listening and discrimination of sounds from the first year of life and then games to encourage imitation and spontaneous production of speech sounds, words and sentences are important for all children if they are to master clear speech. Attention to good feeding, chewing and breathing patterns and encouraging control over fine movement of the muscles of the face, mouth and tongue will also help. The whole range of usual approaches to speech and language therapy may be useful and their application for children with Down syndrome across the age range is well described by Kumin (1994). However, I wish to focus on language learning and to consider the following:

1. The general conclusion that can be drawn from the evidence, which is that learning language from listening is going to be especially difficult for children with Down syndrome so that making it visual may help. Signing and reading are both visual forms of language that may be effective as augmentative systems.
2. The possibility that improving auditory short-term memory function will accelerate language learning, particularly grammar.

At the University of Portsmouth, my research colleagues and I have conducted research on the reading and memory issues over a number of years. This programme of work is ongoing and I will outline our key findings to date after considering signing.

Signing

Practitioners have advocated the use of augmentative signing with babies with Down syndrome since the early 1980s and evidence for its effectiveness has accumulated slowly (e.g. Foreman and Crews 1998; Miller 1995, et al.). It can help in a number of ways. If parents sign as they speak, they make sure the baby is looking, the sign holds the baby's attention and it gives an added clue to the meaning of the words. Parents are also likely to stress the words they are signing. In other words, signing may help to structure more effective language learning situations. For infants, it can increase their productive vocabularies as they can usually sign words before being able to say them. This will reduce frustration and increase communication opportunities. However, it is essential to keep up activities to encourage sound and speech production alongside the use of signing, if children are to move into using spoken words as early as possible. In our experience, most children are able to drop the use of sign slowly from around five years of age, though they should not be discouraged from using sign at any age as a repair strategy when their speech is not understood. The potential ways in which signing may assist speech and language skills in people with Down syndrome warrants more sophisticated analysis than we have available to date as one study illustrated that the speech clarity of adults with Down syndrome improved when they signed as they spoke (Powell and Clibbens 1994). I have heard many individual case examples from parents and practitioners which indicate that: signing often helps the child with Down syndrome find the word and speak more clearly; signs for sounds have helped production of initial and end sounds in words and signs can help to teach grammar.

Reading

We have been studying the reading abilities of children with Down syndrome since 1980. For the first ten years we collected case study data on a number of children and we have published this information on a number of occasions (eg, Buckley 1985, 1995; Buckley and Bird 1993; Buckley et al. 1996). My interest in reading was the result of a letter from a father, Leslie Duffen, describing the progress of his daughter, Sarah. Leslie informed me that Sarah had been able to begin to learn to read from the age of three years and that she had achieved a high level of functional literacy. He also thought that her reading ability had led to her having better speech and language skills than most children with Down syndrome of her age. Leslie felt sure that other children with Down syndrome might benefit in the same ways from early reading instruction and was hoping to interest me in starting some research. He succeeded and our case study data has confirmed his hypotheses. We have worked with many children who have the ability to learn sight vocabularies from as early as two years and four months of age. Most have proceeded to achieve functional levels of reading and writing abilities i.e. above eight year reading ages for reading, and spelling abilities with good comprehension provided that they continue to receive appropriate instruction. Teachers need to be able to adapt the teaching of reading to take account of the child's level of language comprehension and then to use reading ability to teach grammar and vocabulary. Like Sarah, our reading children have better language and they usually have clearer speech.

Not all children will be early readers. We try teaching a sight vocabulary once a child has a comprehension vocabulary of 40 to 50 words and can play matching, selecting and naming games with pictures (eg, picture lotto). We then introduce family names by playing the same matching, selecting and naming games with words. At the same time we make individual books for the child using family photographs, so that the words being learned can be used in meaningful context as we proceed. If the child learns to read the names, we then teach some verbs, nouns and adjectives so that we can begin to build two and three word phrases such as 'mummy sleeping', 'daddy gone', 'big bus', 'Jenny eat cake', 'big black dog' and so on. The sentence structures will start at the level of the child's comprehension and then build from there to teach grammar as well as vocabulary.

If the child is not interested in reading, at the 50 word vocabulary comprehension stage we continue with all the usual language teaching activities and we would try picture symbol systems as visual supports for words and sentence building. We would continue to make and read simple books and play word lottos as most children will be able to learn a sight vocabulary by five years of age. It is essential to keep the activities meaningful and fun for the child. By making individual books about the child's own family, friends and experiences we make comprehension easy and ensure we are teaching language that the child will be able to use to talk about his everyday world at home and at school.

Once a child is confidently reading some 50 words and can read simple sentences with comprehension, then we begin to teach phonics starting with initial consonants in words the child can already read. We find that many children are able to learn letter sounds using the same activities as the other children in their mainstream classes. However, it takes several years of reading instruction to learn to decode a new word in a sentence by 'sounding' it out letter by letter and to be able to spell by thinking how the word sounds to find the letters. When they can do this they have become 'alphabetic' readers and while they are still relying on visual memory for reading and spelling they are 'logographic' readers. These stages have been documented in all beginning readers (see Gathercole and Baddeley 1993 for an overview of reading acquisition in typically developing children).

Longitudinal studies

While many children with Down syndrome were in special schools it was difficult for us to study reading, as it was not a priority on the curriculum - if, indeed, it was taught at all. As we have succeeded in increasing the number of children being educated in mainstream schools over the past ten years, we are now able to study the literacy development of representative samples of children over time and have had one such study ongoing since 1994. We have 24 children with Down syndrome in this study and we are comparing their reading progress with that of a group of their mainstream peers matched for reading age and a group of average readers. We are charting their reading progress, language and memory skills over time. Over the first two years, the children with Down syndrome made as much progress as the reading matched group on reading, so are within the range of readers in their school. They are relying more on visual, logographic strategies to keep up this reading progress and becoming alphabetic more slowly. However, those with reading ages over seven years are slowly mastering the use of phonics for reading and spelling and becoming alphabetic, just like other children, despite their hearing and auditory processing difficulties (Byrne, MacDonald and Buckley, in preparation). We are currently exploring the links between their alphabetic skills and their phonological awareness (Fletcher et al. in preparation). We are not yet able to see any clear pattern of causal relationships between reading, language and memory development as suggested by some of our earlier data (see below) but continue to monitor progress each year (Byrne, Buckley, MacDonald and Bird, in preparation).

Short-term memory, reading, and language

Our attention was drawn to the limited auditory short-term memory spans of children and teenagers with Down syndrome by the work of Mackenzie and Hulme in 1987. In 1990 we began to plan an intervention study to see if we could teach children with Down syndrome to improve their memory function. We evaluated two strategies, rehearsal and organization, which we know are effective memory strategies that typically developing children are able to use in their early school years. In the rehearsal training, children were taught to learn lists of items by rehearsing them aloud and in order. Using picture materials children named and then recalled pictures, starting with one item, then two and so on until they reached their limit. In the organization training the children were taught to group items into categories to help to remember them.

The children were able to use both strategies and training significantly improved both visual and auditory short-term spans (Broadley et al. 1994). The trained children also showed a significant gain in comprehension of grammar in the year compared with children who did not take part in the memory training.

However, as we followed the children over time, the improvement in memory function did not appear to be sustained when we looked at the group data. By three years after training, the children's memory spans appeared to be no better than those of a comparison group who had not done the training (Laws, MacDonald et al. 1995). However, closer inspection of the data revealed a different story, as can be seen in Table 9.1. If the children were divided into those who were able to score on a reading test and those who could not, then the data showed that the readers had continued to build on the improved memory span gained by training but the nonreaders had lost the improvement over time. We then looked back at all the assessment data collected on these children at the start of the study four years earlier. This is set out in Table 9.2. There were no significant differences between the two groups in 1991 on nonverbal mental ability (Raven's Coloured Matrices (RCM)), vocabulary comprehension (British Picture Vocabulary (BPVS)), grammar comprehension (Test for Reception of Grammar (TROG)), or on auditory or visual short-term span. In 1995, both groups of children had made similar progress on the nonverbal mental ability task and both groups made the same progress with memory spans after the training. However, by 1995 the reading group is significantly ahead on the vocabulary, grammar and memory measures. The readers in the comparison group who did not do the memory training also had better auditory and visual short-term memory spans suggesting that the effect in the trained group is due to reading (Laws, Buckley et al. 1995).

Table 9.1 The influence of reading instruction on memory function over time

Auditory memory span				
	Pre-training Oct 1991	Post-training June 1992	8 months later March 1993	3 years later June 1995
Nonreaders	1.43 (.37)	2.14 (.42)	2.10 (.25)	1.62 (.62)
Readers	1.48 (.54)	2.05 (.56)	2.43 (.90)	2.62 (.35)
Visual memory span				
	Pre-training Oct 1991	Post-training June 1992	8 months later March 1993	3 years later June 1995
Nonreaders	1.48 (.42)	3.24 (.63)	3.00 (1.10)	1.89 (.50)
Readers	1.48 (.46)	3.38 (.93)	3.71 (1.18)	2.76 (.25)

Mean short-term auditory and visual memory scores for readers and nonreaders (standard deviations in parentheses) adapted with permission from Laws, Buckley et al. 1995.

Table 9.2 The influence of reading instruction on language and memory development

Cognitive measures	October 1991		July 1995	
	Readers (N=7)	Nonreaders (N=7)	Readers (N=7)	Nonreaders (N=7)
Matrices	2.83 (2.31)	1.68 (.52)	12.83 (7.0)*	11.17 (6.31)*
BPVS	7.43 (2.99)	5.57 (2.15)	11.71 (2.43)	6.86 (3.29)
TROG	3.71 (2.14)	2.14 (1.22)	6.57 (2.37)	2.86 (2.61)
Auditory memory	1.48 (.54)	1.43 (.37)	2.62 (.36)	1.62 (.62)
Visual memory	1.48 (.42)	1.48 (.46)	2.76 (.25)*	1.89 (.50)
		(*N=6)		

Mean matrices, language and memory scores for readers and nonreaders in 1991 and 1995 (with standard deviations in parentheses) adapted with permission from Laws, Buckley et al. 1995.

Finally, we were aware that in the trained group, the readers were all in mainstream schools and the nonreaders in special schools so we looked at data on a similar age group of children from all those in special schools assessed in 1991 and divided them into readers and nonreaders. This is set out in Table 9.3 and we see the same pattern of advantage to the readers. Taken together all this data is pointing to the significant effect that reading will have on the other cognitive skills for children with Down syndrome. As the same beneficial effects of progress with reading on speech, language and memory skills are reported in typically developing children (see longitudinal studies reported in Gathercole and Baddeley 1993), it seems that these cognitive skills are building and supporting one another in the same way in children with Down syndrome.

Table 9.3 Readers and nonreaders in special schools

	Readers (N=17)	Nonreaders (N=17)	Difference
Vocabulary (BPVS)	11.29 (3.90)	7.71 (2.02)	3.58 (p=.007)
Grammar (TROG)	6.82 (2.27)	3.51 (1.23)	3.31 (p=.000)
Auditory memory	2.45 (.42)	1.63 (.37)	.82 (p=.000)
Visual memory	2.37 (.44)	1.65 (.53)	.72 (p=.001)

Language and memory measures for special school readers and nonreaders (standard deviations in parentheses) adapted with permission from Laws, Buckley et al. 1995.

Conclusions

I have endeavoured to illustrate that speech and language skills are central in the development of cognitive abilities and that therefore every effort should be made to help children with Down syndrome to overcome the difficulties that delay and disrupt their progress in this area. In addition to the usual range of effective speech and language interventions I have emphasized the importance of visual supports for learning, particularly signing and reading.

I have presented evidence to support the proposal that reading instruction will not only lead to useful levels of functional literacy for a majority of children, but also improve speech, language and short-term memory skills.

References

Broadley I, MacDonald J, Buckley SJ (1994) Are children with Down's syndrome able to maintain skills learned from a short-term memory training programme? Down's Syndrome: Research and Practice 2: 116-22.

Buckley SJ (1985) Attaining basic educational skills: reading, writing and number. In Lane D, Stratford B (eds) Current approaches to Down's syndrome. Eastbourne: Holt, Rinehart and Winston. pp. 315-43.

Buckley SJ (1993) Developing the speech and language skills of teenagers with Down's syndrome. Down's Syndrome: Research and Practice 1: 63-71.

Buckley SJ (1995a) Increasing the conversational utterance length of teenagers with Down's syndrome. Down's Syndrome: Research and Practice 3: 110-16.

Buckley SJ (1995b) Teaching children with Down syndrome to read and write. In Nadel L, Buckley SJ (1998) Speech, language and literacy in children with Down syndrome. Invited review. The International Journal of Disability, Development and Education. (In press.)

Rosenthal D (eds) Down syndrome: Living and Learning in the Community. New York: Wiley-Liss. pp. 158-69.

Buckley S J, Bird G (1993) Teaching children with Down syndrome to read. Down Syndrome: Research and Practice 1: 34-41.

Buckley SJ, Bird G, Byrne A (1996) Reading acquisition by young children with Down syndrome. In Stratford B, Gunn P(eds) New Approaches to Down Syndrome. London: Cassell. pp. 268-79.

Byrne A, Buckley S, MacDonald J, Bird, G (1998a) A four-year longitudinal study of reading development in children with Down syndrome: Progress and variability. (In preparation.)

Byrne A, MacDonald J, Buckley S (1998b) The development of reading strategies over time for children with Down syndrome and their mainstream peers. (In preparation.)

Chapman RS (1995) Language development in children and adults with Down syndrome. In Fletcher P, MacWhinney B (eds) Handbook of Child Language. Oxford: Blackwell Scientific. pp. 641-63.

Chapman RS (1997a) Language development. In Pueschel SM, Sustrova M (eds) Adolescents with Down Syndrome. Baltimore, MD: Brookes. pp. 99-110.

Chapman RS (1997b) Language development in children and adolescents with Down syndrome. Mental Retardation and Developmental Disabilities Research Reviews 3: 307-12.

Fletcher H, Byrne A, Buckley SJ (1998) Phonological awareness in readers with Down syndrome. (In preparation.)

Foreman P, Crews G (1998) Using augmentative communication with infants and young children with Down syndrome. Down Syndrome: Research and Practice 5, 1: 16-25.

Fowler A (1995) Linguistic variability in persons with Down syndrome: research and implications. In Nadel L, Rosenthal D (eds) Down Syndrome: Living and Learning in the Community. New York: Wiley-Liss. pp. 121-31.

Gathercole SE (1998) The development of memory. Journal of Child Psychology and Psychiatry 39: 3-27.

Gathercole SE, Baddeley AD(1993) Working Memory and Language. Hove: Lawrence Erlbaum.

Kumin L (1994) Communication Skills in Children with Down Syndrome: A Guide for Parents. New York: Woodbine House.

Laws G, Buckley SJ, Bird G, MacDonald J, Broadley I (1995) The influence of reading instruction on language and memory development in children with Down's syndrome. Down's Syndrome: Research and Practice 3: 59-64.

Laws G, MacDonald J, Broadley I (1995) Long-term maintenance of memory skills taught to children with Down's syndrome. Down's Syndrome: Research and Practice 3: 103-9.

Mackenzie S, Hulme C (1987) Memory span development in Down's syndrome, severely subnormal and normal subjects. Cognitive Neuropsychology 4: 303-19.

Mackenzie S, Hulme C (1992) Working Memory and Severe Learning Difficulties. Hove: Lawrence Erlbaum.

Marcell MM (1995) Relationships between hearing and auditory cognition in Down's syndrome youth. Down's Syndrome: Research and Practice 3: 75-91.

Miller JF (1988) The developmental asynchrony of language development in children with Down syndrome. In Nadel L (ed) The Psychobiology of Down Syndrome. Cambridge, MA: MIT Press. pp. 167-98.

Miller JF, Leddy M, Miolo G et al. (1995) The development of early learning skills in children with Down syndrome. In Nadel L, Rosenthal D (eds) Down Syndrome: Living and Learning in the Community. New York: Wiley-Liss. pp. 115-21.

Powell G, Clibbens J (1994) Actions speak louder than words: signing and speech intelligibility in adults with Down's syndrome. Down's Syndrome: Research and Practice 2: 127-9.

Rondal J (1995) Exceptional Language Development in Down Syndrome. Cambridge: Cambridge University Press.

Stoel-Gammon C (1997) Phonological development in Down syndrome. Mental Retardation and Developmental Disabilities Research Reviews 3: 300-6.

Chapter 10
Temperament in Children with Down Syndrome

MARJORIE BEEGHLY

Children with Down syndrome have often been portrayed as happy, affectionate, and mild individuals with 'easy' temperaments (Gibbs and Thorpe 1983; Gibson 1978). In this chapter, the empirical evidence for this stereotype will be reviewed and critically evaluated. This review will be limited to studies using parent-report temperament inventories, as these studies comprise the bulk of this research. Particular emphasis will be placed on troubling methodological issues in this literature that confound interpretation and limit generalizability. A consideration of these issues will make it clear that we still know very little about the temperament characteristics of children with Down syndrome.

Children's temperament is important to evaluate because it has social and developmental consequences. Variations in temperament influence the frequency and the quality of children's social interactions with family members, peers, and teachers (Greenberg and Field 1983; Huntington and Simeonsson 1993; Kagan et al. 1994; Keogh and Burstein 1988). Child temperament is also related to parental adaptation, childrearing practices, and family climate (Gunn and Berry 1985a; Marcovitch et al. 1987; Pueschel and Myers 1994; Seifer and Schiller 1995; Turner et al. 1991). In turn, these social variables affect the child's own development in a transactional manner (Chess 1990; Sameroff and Fiese 1990; Thomas and Chess 1989). For example, variations in child temperament predict children's success in school (Keogh 1994; Martin 1988, 1994; Orth and Martin 1994).

Temperament also affects the well-being of developmentally delayed children (Huntington and Simeonsson 1993). Zigler and colleagues (eg, Zigler and Hodapp 1991) demonstrated that temperament and personality factors contribute to the adaptive functioning and life success of children with the cultural-familial type of mental retardation. Similar findings have been reported for other groups of developmentally delayed children, including children with Down syndrome (Dykens et al. 1994; Goldberg and Marcovitch 1989; Lewis 1992; Martin 1992; Richards 1986).

111

Following a brief definition of 'temperament', three primary questions will be addressed:

1. Do the temperamental characteristics of children with Down syndrome differ significantly from those of normally developing children of similar age or mental abilities?
2. Is there evidence for a unique temperament profile for children with Down syndrome? That is, do the temperamental characteristics of these children differ from those reported for other groups of developmentally delayed children?
3. Can the temperament characteristics of children with Down syndrome be modified by age or environmental factors, as is the case for typically developing children (Belsky et al. 1991; Garrison and Earls 1987)?

Possible directions for future research and educational implications for children with Down syndrome will also be considered.

Definition of Temperament

'Temperament' in this chapter refers to the characteristic style or manner with which persons engage their world (Ganiban et al. 1990). Individual differences in temperament are well documented for normally developing children (Kohnstamm et al. 1989). For instance, children vary in how active they are, how quickly and intensely they react to stimulation, and how cheerful or irritable they are (Bates 1989; Rothbart 1981). Children also differ in their tendency to approach or withdraw from unfamiliar persons or events (Kagan et al. 1994).

Although much controversy exists concerning the nature of temperament (Kohnstamm et al. 1989), most theorists agree that temperament is constitutionally based, appears early in life, and is relatively stable throughout childhood (Matheny et al. 1984; Plomin 1990). However, there is considerable disagreement regarding the degree to which temperament can be modified by development or environmental factors (Goldsmith and Campos 1982). Given that temperament has genetic underpinnings, it is plausible that children with Down syndrome, with their common chromosomal abnormalities, have unique temperamental profiles. If so, this would have important implications for the design and implementation of educational and intervention programmes for these children. However, as will be seen, the empirical evidence supporting this possibility is weak (Goldberg and Marcovitch 1989).

Measurement of Temperament

Most investigators have relied on parent-report inventories to measure variations in child temperament. Although the specific inventories used in different studies vary, there is considerable convergence across different instruments in what is measured. The most commonly assessed dimensions are *emotionality*, *sociability*, and *activity* (Goldsmith et al. 1991; Kohnstamm et al. 1989).

Many extant parent-report temperament inventories (including many used in the Down syndrome literature) were inspired by a landmark temperament research project conducted by Alexander Thomas, Stella Chess and colleagues: the New York Longitudinal Study (Thomas and Chess 1977). In that project, individual differences among children were documented on the following nine dimensions (ratings) of temperament: Activity level; Approach/withdrawal (sociability); Rhythmicity (regularity of biological and behavioural functions such as sleep); Adaptability; Threshold to response; Intensity of response; Mood; Distractibility; and Persistence (see eg, Carey and McDevitt 1978).

Four temperament categories are often derived from these nine temperament ratings: Easy; Intermediate; Difficult; and Slow to Warm Up. The two temperament categories assessed most often in the Down syndrome literature are the Easy and Difficult categories. The Easy category includes children who are highly rhythmic, adaptable, sociable, and cheerful, and only mildly intense. In contrast, children categorized as Difficult are low in rhythmicity, low in adaptability, withdrawing, negative, and intense.

Methodological Issues

As in the normative literature, studies of temperament in children with Down syndrome vary markedly in methodology, making it difficult to generalize findings across studies. One major problem is that different investigators have utilized different comparison groups. Children with Down syndrome have been compared to: (a) their normally developing siblings (eg, Gunn and Berry 1985a; Pueschel and Myers 1994); (b) published age norms (Gunn and Berry 1985b; Gunn and Cuskelly 1991; Marcovitch et al. 1986); (c) age-matched, normally developing children (eg, Ratekin 1996; Rothbart and Hanson 1983); (d) mental-age-matched, normally developing children (eg, Bridges and Cicchetti 1982; Vaughn et al. 1994); (e) and/or other types of developmentally delayed children (eg, Marcovitch et al. 1986, 1987). Although each type of comparison group provides valuable information, each yields a different pattern of results, making generalization of findings difficult. In general, group differences are more likely to be significant when children with Down syndrome are compared to *age norms* or *age-matched* normally developing children (Goldberg and Marcovitch 1989; Ratekin 1996) than when *mental-age-matched* controls are used (eg, Baron 1972; Vaughn et al. 1994). However, this is not consistently true (eg, Huntington and Simeonsson 1987).

Another methodological complication is that the age of children being evaluated varies widely across studies. This is problematic because the expression of temperament changes as children grow older (Belsky et al. 1991; Garrison and Earls 1987; Gunn et al. 1983; Vaughn et al. 1994). In addition, parent-report instruments often include different items for different age groups (eg, Bates and Bayles 1984; Ratekin 1996; Vaughn et al. 1994), confounding interpretation.

A third difficulty concerns the almost exclusive use of parent-report temperament inventories in this literature, without the additional use of direct observations of child behaviour (see Gil et al. 1996, for an exception). Although these instruments typically have good internal statistical properties and are convenient and economical to use, they have several drawbacks. One of the most serious is their questionable validity (Sanson et al. 1990; Seifer et al. 1994; Vaughn 1986).

For instance, different informants (eg, mother, father, teacher) rating the same child do not typically agree with each other (Marcovitch et al. 1986; Seifer et al. 1994). Moreover, temperament ratings do not necessarily reflect the child's *actual* behaviour (Seifer and Sameroff 1986; Vaughn 1986) and are not always stable over time (Belsky et al. 1991; Stifter and Fox 1990). Furthermore, parents' temperament ratings are related to nonchild factors such as socioeconomic status, parental adaptation, and child rearing practices (Marcovitch et al. 1987; Seifer and Sameroff 1986; Vaughn et al. 1987). Thus, it is unclear what these instruments are actually measuring.

In addition, different investigators of child temperament tend to use different temperament measures, such as temperament *categories* (Easy, Difficult), ratings (eg, Distractibility), or *parental impressions* measures. Measurement differences are problematic because they affect the type and significance of the results obtained (Goldberg and Marcovitch 1989; Ratekin 1996). In general, significant findings are more likely to be obtained when ratings of temperament dimensions are used. Even so, the *specific* temperament dimensions that distinguish children with Down syndrome from other children differ from study to study. The most reliably reported group differences are for Persistence and Approach (Bridges and Cicchetti 1982; Gunn and Berry 1985b; Gunn and Cuskelly 1991; Huntington and Simeonsson 1987; Marcovitch et al. 1986; Pueschel and Myers 1994; Ratekin 1996). Adults tend to perceive children with Down syndrome as less persistent than normally developing children, and as either more or less sociable, depending on the age of the children under study (Goldberg and Marcovitch 1989).

Two Illustrative Studies

To illustrate some of the methodological differences in this literature, two recent studies of temperament in children with Down syndrome will be presented. Critically, both studies were methodologically sound and utilized appropriate multivariate statistical techniques.

The first study is a large cross-sectional study of temperament in children with Down syndrome (Ratekin 1996). In this study, the maternal temperament ratings of 191 children with Down syndrome were compared with those made for 388 normally developing, age-matched children. The children were divided into four age groups for analysis: infants, toddlers, preschoolers, and early school-aged children. Mothers completed the short-form version of the Parent Temperament Questionnaire (PTQ; Keogh et al. 1982), which assesses similar temperament dimensions as in the New York Longitudinal Study (Thomas and Chess 1977) but uses the same items for all age groups.

On average, the children with Down syndrome were rated as being significantly less persistent, more sociable, more distractible, and more positive in mood than the age-matched normally developing children. Significant age-related changes were also found for both the children with Down syndrome and the comparison children on three temperament dimensions: Mood, Distractibility, and Intensity. Mood and Distractibility were highest in infancy, whereas Intensity was lowest.

Interestingly, the age effect for Mood was qualified by a significant group by age interaction effect. Compared with their age-matched, normally developing counterparts, infants with Down syndrome were rated *lower* in positive mood, whereas older children with Down syndrome were rated higher in positive mood. These findings suggest that, during infancy, children with Down syndrome are perceived as more negative or difficult than age-matched normally developing infants. However, with increasing child age, this trend reverses itself. Ratekin speculated that these data may provide support for the 'easy' stereotype for *older* children with Down syndrome. Similar findings were reported more than a decade ago for children with Down syndrome by Gunn et al. (1983) and for normally developing children by McDevitt and Carey (1978).

The second study is a smaller longitudinal study of 32 infants and toddlers with Down syndrome and 44 mental-age-matched normally developing infants (Vaughn et al. 1994). In this study, mothers completed the Toddler Temperament Scales (TTS; Fullard et al. 1984), which were derived from the New York Longitudinal Study, or the Bates Infant/Child Characteristics Questionnaire (ICQ; Bates and Bayles 1984) at two time points between 12 and 36 months of age. The average mental ages of the study children at Time 1 and Time 2 were 16 and 23 months, respectively.

In contrast to Ratekin's findings, there were *no* significant group differences on the TTS. However, on the Bates ICQ, the children with Down syndrome differed from controls on two temperament dimensions: Unstoppable and Dependent. Additionally, age-related changes in child temperament were reported. In both the Down syndrome and comparison samples, maternal ratings of child difficulty decreased significantly from infancy to toddlerhood. However, in contrast to Ratekin's findings, there were no significant group differences in child difficulty at either time period. These findings suggest that child age influences maternal perceptions of child temperament.

The discrepant findings in Ratekin's and Vaughn's studies are puzzling until one acknowledges the striking methodological differences between them. For instance, Ratekin's study was cross-sectional and involved a wide age range of children, whereas Vaughn et al.'s study was longitudinal and included only infants and toddlers. Moreover, in Ratekin's study, the Down syndrome and normally developing groups were age-matched, whereas in Vaughn et al.'s study, groups were matched for cognitive ability. Another critical difference was that different parent-report instruments were used in the two studies. These methodological differences preclude direct comparisons of the two studies. Unfortunately, these differences are characteristic of those in many studies in this literature.

A Unique Temperament Profile?

Is there any evidence that children with Down syndrome exhibit a unique temperament profile? Several investigators have attempted to answer this question by comparing temperament ratings made for children with Down syndrome with those made for other groups of developmentally delayed children. In one recent study, Marcovitch et al. (1987) compared maternal temperament ratings made for three types of developmentally delayed preschoolers (M age = 39 months): children with Down syndrome, children with neurological problems, and children with unexplained delays. The three diagnostic groups differed significantly in Activity level, Approach/withdrawal, and Distractibility. Contrary to the existing folklore, however, the children with Down syndrome were not always at the 'easy' end of the continuum on these ratings. Moreover, findings varied with the type of measure used.

Further comparative research is needed to replicate and elaborate these findings.

Caution

Caution is warranted in interpreting these findings and others like it in this literature. Typically, the group differences reported are small. Often, the group means are smaller in magnitude than the standard deviations. This suggests that individual children with Down syndrome and comparison children *vary* on specific dimensions of temperament. Hence, while the group differences reported in this literature are significant, they say little about the temperament profiles of individual children.

Individuality and Down Syndrome: A Case Study

Even when significant group differences are reported, many investigators concur that children with Down syndrome exhibit a range of temperament characteristics (Huntington and Simeonsson 1993). To illustrate this individuality, a case study of five-year-old twin girls with Down syndrome will be presented. The twins currently attend a mainstream kindergarten in the greater Boston metropolitan area. Although the twins are both happy and positive children, their parents and teachers agree that each has a unique personality. One twin is described as being a leader and a 'spitfire' who reacts intensely to stimulation with either heightened positive or negative affect. She is also described as being independent and somewhat a 'loner' socially. In contrast, the second twin is described as being highly sociable, dependent, and a 'follower', with more even-keeled emotionality. This case study illustrates that children with Down syndrome may exhibit a wide range of temperament traits, despite their common chromosomal abnormalities and neurodevelopmental processes.

Environmental Influences

It is well documented in normative samples that environmental factors such as caregiving style and social context influence the expression of child temperament. For example, Kagan et al. (1994) showed that parents can encourage extremely shy children to become less inhibited over time. Similarly, van den Boom (1994) demonstrated that positive changes in mothers' sensitive caregiving resulted in higher levels of sociability and less crying in their infants. Moreover, differences in social contexts can affect the expression of temperament. For example, children are generally more active and exuberant on the playground than in a classroom.

Very few studies have evaluated environmental influences on the expression of temperament in children with Down syndrome. In one exception, Greenberg and Field (1983) found that social context influenced maternal temperament ratings of a mixed group of handicapped children, including children with Down syndrome. In that study, more 'difficult' ratings were assigned during classroom play than during dyadic interactions. In other research, Pueschel and Myers (1994) evaluated maternal and teacher temperament ratings of children with Down syndrome and their normally developing siblings. Although parents and teachers both rated children with Down syndrome as less persistent than age-norms, only the teachers rated the children with Down syndrome as more distractible. This finding may reflect different constraints on child attention in the home and school settings.

Pueschel and Myers also reported that family climate factors such as expressiveness and control were significantly related to child temperament ratings. For instance, familial expressiveness was positively correlated with child persistence and negatively correlated with child activity level. These findings need to be replicated with more comprehensive measurement of children's social environments.

Conclusions

Methodological differences among studies of temperament in children with Down syndrome abound. These differences limit the interpretation and generalizability of findings in this literature. Nevertheless, several tentative conclusions can be made regarding the temperament characteristics of children with Down syndrome, as follows.

First, most researchers agree that individual children with Down syndrome exhibit a broad range of temperament characteristics. Although some find significant differences in temperament between Down syndrome and other groups, the magnitude of these differences is typically small, and within-group variation is high. Thus, stereotyped perceptions of temperament in children with Down syndrome are not necessarily accurate or helpful.

Second, although further research is needed, there is some evidence that children with Down syndrome *as a group* may exhibit common temperament features. Across studies, the most reliably reported temperament differences for these children are for Persistence and Approach. In addition, mothers appear to perceive their *older* children with Down syndrome as temperamentally 'easier' than same-aged normally developing children, on average. However, this stereotype does not apparently hold for infants with Down syndrome. Without direct behaviour observations, it is impossible to know whether these differences reflect actual changes in children's behaviour over time or merely changes in maternal adaptation. Of note, significant differences have been reported in these children's socioaffective, attentional, and information processing competencies (eg, Cicchetti and Beeghly 1990; Cicchetti et al. 1991; Green et al. 1989; Kasari et al. 1990; Kopp and Recchia 1990; Lewis 1992; MacTurk and Vietze 1985; Thompson et al. 1985). Such neurodevelopmental differences may indeed influence adults' perceptions of these children.

Third, similar age-related changes in temperament have been observed for both children with Down syndrome and normally developing children. This suggests that the sequence of temperament development for children with Down syndrome is broadly similar to that reported for normally developing children. However, the methodological differences among studies preclude any firm conclusions.

Future Research Directions

To overcome some of the methodological difficulties in this literature, future research should aim towards establishing a normative database integrating *both* personality and behavioural characteristics of children with Down syndrome and other groups of developmentally delayed children. This database should include the following: large, longitudinal samples; multiple comparison groups (eg, both age-matched and mental-age-matched groups of typical children; other groups of developmentally delayed children); repeated behavioural observations of children in multiple social contexts (including school settings); and reports from multiple informants (eg, parents, teachers). The rich, detailed data generated by this approach will necessitate the use of multivariate statistical analyses.

In addition, further study of the effect of the social environment on children's temperament and personality development is needed. In this research, investigators should employ multiple measures of children's social contexts, including measures of parent and familial adaptation, peer relations, school functioning, and demographic/cultural factors.

Educational and Clinical Implications

Educational and intervention programmes that consider temperament are likely to benefit children with Down syndrome. Keogh (1994), Martin (1988, 1994; Orth and Martin 1994) and others have shown that variations in children's temperament are important predictors of their success in school. Because children with Down syndrome may differ from normally developing children on specific temperament dimensions (eg, Persistence, Distractibility) known to influence school functioning, programmes that accommodate these differences may facilitate these children's adaptation to school (Ratekin 1996). In addition, educational and community programmes that promote increased direct contact of children with Down syndrome with typical children and adults may help reduce harmful stereotypical perceptions of children with Down syndrome (Wishart and Johnston 1990).

Ultimately, temperament is related to quality of life. Researchers, clinicians, and educators are becoming increasingly aware that social and personality factors, including temperament, contribute to children's life success and happiness. Although further research is needed, the empirical evidence clearly indicates that children with Down syndrome are unique individuals. Through a better understanding of these children's temperamental characteristics and the factors that influence them, families, communities and society will be better able to support the positive development of children and young people with Down syndrome. With their diverse personalities and gifts, these individuals truly have much to offer the world.

Acknowledgements

I am grateful to Glenn K Wasek for his thoughtful conceptual input and to Erik Holling and Henrietta Kernan for their valuable assistance with the preparation of this manuscript.

References

Baron S (1972) Temperament profile of children with Down syndrome. Developmental Medicine and Child Neurology 14: 640-3.

Bates JE (1989) Applications of temperament concepts. In Kohnstamm GA, Bates JE, Rothbart MK (eds) Temperament in Childhood. New York: Wiley. pp. 321-55.

Bates JE, Bayles K (1984) Objective and subjective components in mothers' perceptions of their children from age 6 months to 3 years. Merrill-Palmer Quarterly 30: 111-29.

Belsky J, Fish M, Isabella R (1991) Continuity and discontinuity in infant negative and positive emotionality. Developmental Psychology 27: 421-31.

Bridges FA, Cicchetti D (1982) Mothers' ratings of the temperament characteristics of Down syndrome infants. Developmental Psychology 18: 238-44.

Carey WB, McDevitt SC (1978) Revision of the Infant Temperament Questionnaire. Pediatrics 61: 735-9.

Chess S (1990) Studies in temperament: a paradigm in psychosocial research. The Yale Journal of Biology and Medicine 63: 313-24.

Cicchetti D, Beeghly M (1990) An organizational approach to the study of Down syndrome: contributions to an integrative theory of development. In Cicchetti D, Beeghly M (eds) Children with Down Syndrome: A Developmental Perspective. New York: Cambridge University Press. pp. 29-62.

Cicchetti D, Ganiban JM, Barnett D (1991) Contributions from the study of high-risk populations to understanding the development of emotion regulation. In Garber J, Dodge KA (eds) The Development of Emotion Regulation Dysregulation. New York: Cambridge University Press. pp. 15-48.

Dykens EM, Hodapp RM, Evans DW (1994) Profiles and development of adaptive behavior in children with Down syndrome. American Journal on Mental Retardation 98: 580-7.

Fullard W, McDevitt S, Carey W (1984) Assessing temperament in one- to three-year-old children. Journal of Pediatric Psychology 9: 205-17.

Ganiban JM, Wagner S, Cicchetti D (1990) Temperament and Down syndrome. In Cicchetti D, Beeghly M (eds) Children with Down Syndrome: A Developmental Perspective. New York: Cambridge University Press. pp. 63-100.

Garrison WT, Earls FJ (1987) Temperament and child psychopathology. Developmental and Clinical Psychology and Psychiatry, Vol. 12. Beverly Hills, CA: Sage.

Gibbs MV, Thorpe JG (1983) Personality stereotype of noninstitutionalized DS children. American Journal of Mental Deficiency 87: 601-5.

Gibson D (1978) Down's Syndrome: The Psychology of Mongolism. New York: Cambridge University Press.

Gil IC, Carnicerio JAC, Lopez JP (1996) Socioaffective development of infants with Down syndrome. In Rondal JA, Perera J, Nadel L, Comblain A (eds) Down's Syndrome: Psychological, Psychobiological, and Socio-educational Perspectives. London: Whurr. pp. 165-77.

Goldberg S, Marcovitch S (1989) Temperament in developmentally disabled children. In Kohnstamm G, Bates J, Rothbart M (eds), Temperament in Childhood. New York: Wiley. pp. 387-403.

Goldsmith HH, Campos JJ (1982) Toward a theory of temperament. In Emde RN, Harmon R (eds) The Development of Attachment and Affiliative Systems. New York: Plenum.

Goldsmith HH, Rieser-Danner LA, Briggs S (1991) Evaluating convergent and discriminant validity of temperament questionnaires for preschoolers, toddlers, and infants. Developmental Psychology 27: 566-79.

Green JM, Dennis J, Bennets LA (1989) Attention disorder in a group of young Down syndrome children. Journal of Mental Deficiency Research 33, 2: 105-22.

Greenberg R, Field T (1983) Temperament ratings of handicapped infants during class-room, mother, and teacher interacions. Journal of Pediatric Psychology 7: 387-405.

Gunn P, Berry P (1985a) Down's syndrome temperament and maternal response to descriptions of child behavior. Developmental Psychology 21: 842-7.

Gunn P, Berry P (1985b) The temperament of Down's syndrome toddlers and their siblings. Journal of Child Psychiatry and Psychiatry and Allied Disciplines 26: 973-9.

Gunn P, Cuskelly M (1991) Down syndrome temperament: The stereotype at middle childhood and adolescence. International Journal of Disability, Development, and Education 38: 59-70.

Gunn P, Berry P, Andrews RJ (1983) The temperament of Down's syndrome toddlers: a research note. Journal of Child Psychology and Psychiatry and Allied Disciplines 24: 601-5.

Huntington GS, Simeonsson RJ (1987) Down's syndrome and toddler temperament. Child: Care, Health, and Development 13: 1-11.

Huntington GS, Simeonsson RJ (1993) Temperament and adaptation in infants and young children with disabilities. Infant Mental Health Journal 14: 49-60.

Kagan J, Snidman N, Arcus D, Reznick JS (1994) Galen's Prophecy: Temperament in Human Nature. New York: Basic Books.

Kasari C, Mundy P, Yirmiya N, Sigman M (1990) Affect and attention in children with Down syndrome. American Journal on Mental Retardation 95: 55-67.

Keogh BK (1994) Temperament and teachers' views of teachability. In Carey WB, McDevitt SC (eds), Prevention and Early Intervention: Individual Differences as Risk Factors for the Mental Health of Children. New York: Brunner/Mazel. pp. 246-54.

Keogh BK, Burstein ND (1988) Relationship of temperament to preschoolers' interactions with peers and teachers. Exceptional Children 54: 456-61.

Keogh BK, Pullis ME, Cadwell J (1982) Teacher Temperament Questionnaire-Short Form. Journal of Educational Measurement 29: 323-9.

Kohnstamm GA, Bates JE, Rothbart M (1989) (eds) Temperament in Childhood. New York: Wiley.

Kopp C B, Recchia SL (1990) The issues of multiple pathways in the development of handicapped children. In Hodapp RM, Burack JA, Zigler E (eds), Issues in the Developmental Approach to Mental Retardation. New York: Cambridge University Press. pp. 272-93.

Lewis M (1992) Individual differences in response to stress. Pediatrics 90: 487-90.

MacTurk R, Vietze P (1985) Exploratory behavior in Down syndrome. Child Development 56: 573-81.

Marcovitch S, Goldberg S, Lojkasek M, MacGregor DL (1987) The concept of difficult temperament in the developmentally disabled preschool child. Journal of Applied Developmental Psychology 8: 151-64.

Marcovitch S, Goldberg, S, MacGregor D, Lojkasek M (1986). Patterns of temperament variation in three groups of developmentally delayed preschool children: mother and father ratings. Developmental and Behavioral Pediatrics 7: 247-52.

Martin RP (1988) Prediction of elementary school achievement from preschool temperament. three studies. School Psychology Review 17: 125-37

Martin RP (1992) Child temperament effects on special education: process and outcomes. Exceptionality: 99-115.

Martin RP (1994) Child temperament and common problems in schooling: Hypotheses about causal connections. Journal of School Psychology 32: 119-45.

Matheny AP, Wilson RS, Nuss SM (1984) Toddler temperament: stability across settings and ages. Child Development 55: 1200-11.

McDevitt SC, Carey WB (1978) The measurement of temperament in three to seven-year-old children. Journal of Child Psychology and Psychiatry 19: 245-53.

Orth LC, Martin RP (1994) Interactive effects of student temperament and instruction method on classroom behavior and achievement. Journal of School Psychology 32: 149-66.

Plomin R (1990) The role of inheritance in behavior. Science 248: 183-8.

Pueschel SM, Myers BA (1994) Environmental and temperament assessments of children with Down syndrome. Journal of Intellectual Disability Research 38: 195-202.

Ratekin C (1996) Temperament in children with Down syndrome. Developmental Disabilities Bulletin 24: 18-32.

Richards NB (1986) Interaction between mothers and infants with Down syndrome: infant characteristics. Topics in Early Childhood Special Education 6: 54-71.

Rothbart MK (1981) Measurement of infant temperament in infancy. Child Development 52: 569-87.

Rothbart M, Hanson MJ (1983) A caregiver report comparison of temperamental characteristics of Down syndrome and normal infants. Developmental Psychology 19: 766-9.

Sameroff AJ, Fiese BH (1990) Transactional regulation and early intervention. In Meisels SJ, Shonkoff JP (eds) Handbook of Early Childhood Intervention. New York: Cambridge University Press. pp. 119-49.

Sanson A, Prior M, Kyrios M (1990) Contamination of measures in temperament research. Merrill-Palmer Quarterly 36: 179-92.

Seifer R, Sameroff AJ (1986) The concept, measurement, and interpretation of temperament in young children: a survey of research issues. Advances in Developmental and Behavioral Pediatrics 7: 1-43

Seifer R, Sameroff AJ, Barrett LC, Krafchuk E (1994). Infant temperament measured by multiple observations and mother report. Child Development 65: 1478-90.

Seifer R, Schiller M (1995) The role of parenting sensitivity, infant temperament, and dyadic interaction in attachment theory and assessment. Monographs of the Society for Research in Child Development 60: 146-74.

Stifter CA, Fox NA (1990) Infant reactivity: physiological correlates of newborn and 5-month temperament. Developmental Psychology 26: 582-8.

Thomas A, Chess S (1977) Temperament and Development. New York: Brunner-Mazel.

Thomas A, Chess S (1989) Temperament and personality. In Kohnstamm GA, Bates JE, Rothbart MK (eds) Temperament in Childhood. New York: Wiley.

Thompson RA, Cicchetti D, Lamb ME, Malkin C (1985) Emotional responses of Down syndrome and normal infants in the Strange Situation: the organization of affective behavior in infants. Developmental Psychology 21: 828-41.

Turner S, Sloper P, Knussen C, Cunningham CC (1991) Factors relating to self-sufficiency in children with Down's syndrome. Journal of Mental Deficiency Research 35: 13-24.

van den Boom DC (1994) The influence of temperament and mothering on attachment and exploration: an experimental manipulation of sensitive responsiveness among lower-class mothers with irritable infants. Child Development 65: 1457-77.

Vaughn BE (1986) The doubtful validity of infant temperament assessments by means of questionnaires like the ITQ. In Kohnstamm GA (ed) Temperament and Development in Infancy and Childhood. Lisse, Netherlands: Swets and Zeitlinger. pp. 35-42.

Vaughn BE, Bradley CF, Joffe LS, Seifer R, Barglow P (1987) Maternal characteristics measured prenatally predict ratings of temperament 'difficulty' on the Carey Infant Temperament Questionnaire. Developmental Psychology 23: 152-61.

Vaughn BE, Contreras J, Seifer R (1994) Short-term longitudinal study of maternal ratings of temperament in samples of children with Down syndrome and normally developing children. American Journal on Mental Retardation 98: 607-18.

Wishart JG, Johnston FH (1990) The effects of experience on attribution of a stereo-typed personality to children with DS. Journal of Mental Deficiency Research 34: 409-20.

Zigler E, Hodapp RM (1991) Behavioral functioning of individuals with mental retarda-tion. Annual Review of Psychology 42: 29-50.

Chapter 11
Intellectual Development in Children with Down Syndrome

ROBERT M HODAPP, DAVID W EVANS AND F LEE GRAY

In the field of mental retardation, intellectual development is a topic that is both old and new. On the one hand, mental retardation has historically been defined by lower levels of intelligence relative to age-mates. Variations within the mental retardation category have also generally relied on IQ scores; hence, the mild-moderate-severe-profound designations that most researchers and practitioners use to characterize functioning in persons with mental retardation. Such historic concerns continue to this very day, as witnessed by debates about what intelligence is, how it should be measured, and what intelligence's relative weight should be in definitions of mental retardation.

In Down syndrome as well, intellectual development is an old and new topic, with many studies over many years. Even 20 years ago, David Gibson (1978) demonstrated that the field knew quite a bit about intellectual development in children with Down syndrome. Compare this situation with all other genetic disorders of mental retardation. In reviews focusing on various areas of behavioural functioning, we have found that Down syndrome features as many behavioural studies as do all of the 750 remaining genetic retardation disorders combined (Hodapp 1996; Hodapp and Dykens 1994).

Looking at the overall picture, then, one might question why researchers should be concerned about intellectual development in children with Down syndrome. But this big picture obscures some major gaps, some unresolved issues that continue to demand our attention. From our perspective, four characteristics make intellectual development an important area of research in children with Down syndrome.

The first and most obvious characteristic is that most such research is *dated*. In perusing Gibson's (1978) book, one finds that research on children's intellectual development stems from the 1920s and 1930s. This topic probably had its heyday in the 1950s and early 1960s. But in recent years, few studies examine intellectual development. From the 1980s and

1990s, very few studies exist concerning certain developmental periods - for example, the middle childhood and adolescent years.

Partly as a result of this aged research base, few studies examine the intellectual development of children with *Down syndrome compared with other persons with mental retardation*. Indeed, the past decade has featured interest in behavioural characteristics of many different genetic disorders. Although there are still too few studies, intellectual development is one area of interest. Yet studies of intellectual development in other retarded groups need to be juxtaposed with similar studies in Down syndrome.

An aged research base leads to another corollary concerning the *mechanisms* of intellectual development. As noted below, several intriguing findings exist concerning both the trajectories and profiles of intelligence in Down syndrome. Why do children with Down syndrome show particular intellectual profiles? Why is it that the pace of development seems to change at specific time-points? Each question receives few answers when a field has inadequately examined intellectual development in children with Down syndrome.

A final problem is more practical. Over the past few years, several researchers have argued for certain *intervention practices* for children with Down syndrome. Researchers have argued that these children make better intellectual and adaptive gains when certain types of interventions are followed, as opposed to others. For the most part, however, such calls have only begun to be linked to existing profiles of intellectual strengths and weaknesses in this syndrome.

In this chapter, we address several of these issues. We use data from earlier published studies and from an ongoing study at the University of New Orleans. The University of New Orleans data consist of the performance of 52 children who were tested as part of another study. Almost all children (49 of 52) were examined using the Stanford-Binet Scales, 4th edition, the newest version of the Stanford-Binet.

Questions About Intelligence in Down Syndrome

In considering intellectual development in children with Down syndrome, two different sets of questions arise. The first concerns rates of development. The question here concerns how fast the child is developing intellectually. Is intellectual development proceeding faster, slower, or unchanged compared with earlier or later ages? A second type of question concerns profiles. As noted below, children with Down syndrome may show specific intellectual strengths and weaknesses. Both rate and profile questions are of theoretical and practical interest in Down syndrome.

Before beginning, it is important to note that any developmental trajectory or profile will not apply to every child with Down syndrome. Indeed, the so-called 'behavioural phenotype' of Down syndrome is probabilistic in nature. To quote a definition advanced by Elisabeth Dykens (1995), a behavioural phenotype in any genetic syndrome 'may best be described as the heightened *probability* or *likelihood* that people with a given syndrome will exhibit certain behavioural or developmental sequelae relative to those without the syndrome' (p. 523). Although most children with Down syndrome will therefore show the syndrome's 'characteristic' trajectories or profiles, such trajectories or profiles will not be present in every child with this syndrome.

Issues of Rates of Development

Given such preliminaries, we can identify four questions concerning rates of intellectual development in children with Down syndrome.

Question 1: Does IQ go down in Down syndrome with increasing chronological age?

Beginning with Gibson's (1978) review, the large majority of studies have shown a gradual slowing in the rate of development for children with Down syndrome. In Carr's (1992) longitudinal study of children in Surrey, England, for example, she found a gradual decline not only during the early childhood years, but also from ages four to eleven years. Similarly in Cunningham's (1987) study of children from Manchester, he found decreasing rates of intellectual development - as shown by decreasing IQ scores - as these children got older.

As Table 11.1 shows, others have also seen this decline over the years. Limiting our review to published studies examining children living at home (some early studies examined institutionalized children), the large majority show IQ declines for children with Down syndrome. Such declines in rates of development seem particularly salient during the earliest years, although some declines may also occur in the middle child-hood years. Both longitudinal and cross-sectional studies demonstrate such declines in rates of development; in our cross-sectional study, this decline seemed more salient when comparing the five to seven age-group versus children of older ages.

Question 2: Are declines seen in children with mental retardation in general?

The second research question puts the first in perspective. If all children with mental retardation slow in their intellectual development over time, such declines may have little to do with Down syndrome. It may simply be that something about retardation in general makes for slowed intellectual development as children get older.

Although one could compare children with Down syndrome with other aetiological groups, at present it seems best to compare intellectual trajec-

Table 11.1 Longitudinal and cross-sectional studies of IQ in Down syndrome

Study	N	<3	3–5	5–7	7–9	9–11	11–13	13–15	15+
				IQ at ages					
Longitudinal									
Carr 1992	54	80	45				37.2		41.9
Cunningham 1987	181	70.9	58.7						
Cross-sectional									
Melyn & White 1973	642	56.9	51.8	46.9	44.8	42.7	35.9	37.7	
Morgan 1979	217	65.8	45.9	41.0	38.3	33.4	26.8		
This study	52			50.7	41.0	38.7	39.6	37.7	41.3

tories of children with Down syndrome with trajectories of children with mixed or nonspecific mental retardation. Table 11.2 reviews some of these IQ studies in children with mixed or nonspecific mental retardation. Although Bernheimer et al. (1997) disagree somewhat, every other study finds a general stability in IQ scores over time for children with mental retardation in general. Granted, some percentage of individual children decline, but by far the general pattern seems one of IQ stability. This stability occurs at all ages from infancy on. In contrast to the slowing developmental rates for children with Down syndrome as they get older, children with mental retardation in general show steady rates of intellectual development over time.

Question 3: Are these slowed rates, or actual losses in development?

A third question concerns losses of actual skills. So far, the evidence concerns losses of IQ, which indicate slowings in the *rate* of intellectual development. But are children with Down syndrome actually losing already-acquired skills? Such does not appear to be the case. Using our cross-sectional findings as a case in point, children with Down syndrome continue developing as they get older, in every area. For example, Stanford-Binet age-equivalent scores show Vocabulary increasing from an average 3.45 years during the 5-10-year-old period, to 4.80 from 10-15 years, to 5.80 after age 15. Age-equivalent scores on other subtests show similar increases.

Question 4: Are declines in rates of development seen in other areas of functioning?

A final rate question concerns what might be called the 'generalizability' of slowings of rates of development in Down syndrome. To what extent do children with Down syndrome slow in other areas of development?

In our cross-sectional study, we also have scores on the Vineland Adaptive Behavior Scales, a widely-used measure of adaptive functioning.

Table 11.2 Longitudinal studies of IQ in children of mixed or nonspecific aetiologies

Study	N	<3	3–5	5–7	7–9	9–11	11–13	13–15	15+
Bernheimer & Keogh 1988	34–37	67.1		71.3		70.3			
Bernheimer, Keogh & Guthrie, 1997	82		72.2	69.6			66.1		
Silverstein 1982	101					65.7	66.4	64.0	
Stavrou 1990 (mild MR)	60				64.7			63.5	63.1

Using Vineland standard scores, we found a close association between children's IQ scores and Vineland Standard Scores on each of the three domains. IQs and the standard scores in Communication, Daily Living Skills, and Socialization correlated at .68, .59, and .68, respectively.

Table 11.3 shows such relations in another way. As before when examining IQ, we see that the Vineland domain standard scores are declining with age. Adaptively as well, children with Down syndrome are declining in their rates of development as they get older. Also as before, children with Down syndrome continue to develop, but at slowed rates over time.

Issues of Intellectual Strengths and Weaknesses

Moving to our second major issue - intellectual profiles - one main question arises.

Question 5: Do children with Down syndrome show intellectual strengths and weaknesses?

In addition to possible deficits in grammar (Fowler 1990) and in expressive as opposed to receptive language (Miller 1992), it does appear that children with Down syndrome show a particular pattern of intellectual strengths and weaknesses. Specifically, even on studies that have ensured that these children have no hearing losses, children with Down syndrome show better abilities on tasks of visual-spatial versus auditory processing.

Table 11.4 shows this relative advantage of visual over auditory processing in three types of studies. First, two studies examined children with Down syndrome on those Kaufman Assessment Battery for Children subtests involving auditory versus visual processing (Hodapp et al. 1992; Pueschel et al. 1987). In both studies, children with Down syndrome performed much higher - by either scaled or age-equivalent scores - on visual versus auditory processing tasks.

A similar type of analysis can be performed using subtests of the Stanford-Binet IV. Here the two subtests involve Bead Memory - a visual short-term memory task - and Memory for Sentences - an auditory short-term memory task. Again, we see a decided advantage of visual over auditory processing in children with Down syndrome, t (42) = 5.49, p <.0001.

Table 11.3 Vineland Standard Scores and age-equivalents with age

Domain	5–10	10–15	15+
A-Standard Scores			
Communication	47.50	38.45	32.31
Daily Living Skills	38.50	24.90	38.46
Socialization	63.31	52.20	42.85
B-age-equivalents (in years)			
Communication	2.63	4.70	5.66
Daily Living Skills	2.80	4.27	6.09
Socialization	3.42	4.90	5.30

A third type of study involves memory span for auditory versus visually presented items. For most typically developing individuals, a 'modality-effect' exists, such that memory for items presented orally is advanced over memory for visually presented items. In Down syndrome, however, children perform about equally in the two modalities. Relative to the performances of typically developing children, then, children with Down syndrome show a visual advantage. In short, it may help to present items visually versus orally.

Overview

From these data, one can conclude two things: that children with Down syndrome slow in their intellectual development as they get older, and that these children have specific strengths in visual as opposed to auditory processing. In both cases, intellectual declines or profiles do not appear in children who are developing normally, nor in children with mixed or non-specific types of mental retardation.

Given these two findings, the obvious question becomes 'why?' Why do children with Down syndrome slow in their rates of intellectual and adaptive development? Why do these children show advantages in visual versus auditory processing?

Unfortunately, at present we do not know. To address the rate issue first, several candidate hypotheses have been proposed, but these are very preliminary. One idea holds that better environments produce higher IQ or other standard scores. 'Environment' here means several things - parents who provide more optimal stimulation or good early intervention programmes.

To date, this idea receives only limited support in Down syndrome. For example, Cunningham (1987) finds that children from higher socio-economic backgrounds do indeed show higher IQs, which may be an effect of either parental 'background genes' or better home environments. Other studies seem mixed (see Hodapp and Zigler 1990 for a review), and this study's data show that the educational levels of fathers are moderately related to children's IQs, $r = .43$, $p < .002$, but the educational levels of mothers are not, $r = .16$, NS.

Table 11.4 Intellectual strengths and weaknesses in Down syndrome

	Visual tasks		Auditory tasks	
K-ABC studies	Hand Movements (scaled score)	Gestalt Closure	# Recall	Word Order
Pueschel et al. 1987 (scaled)	3.15	4.55	2.35	1.70
Hodapp et al. 1992 (age-equivs)	5.58 (years)	5.40	3.18	3.75
Stanford-Binet IV study	Bead Memory		Memory for Sentences	
This study	3.89 (years)		3.08	
Number of items recalled	Visually presented		Auditorally presented	
	Non-MR	Down syndrome	Non-MR	Down syndrome
Digit Span Studies				
McDade & Adler 1980	2.10	2.10	3.50	2.10
Marcell & Armstrong 1982	2.90	2.45	3.92	2.43

In the same way, some have argued that early intervention may alleviate the slowing developmental rates in children with Down syndrome. But although many studies show short-term IQ gains in children due to early intervention, early intervention has yet to show long-term effects in Down syndrome. To quote Cunningham (1987), 'no support was found for the hypothesis that the early intervention would have long-term benefits reflected in measures of child development' (p. 178).

For now, the best possibilities accounting for developmental slowings might be task-demands, possibly involving the beginnings of language and, possibly, of certain sensorimotor skills (Dunst 1988), or age-related slowings due to (unspecified) brain changes (Dykens et al. 1994; Gibson 1966). Such task- and age-related slowings demand more attention than either has so far received.

When considering profiles of intellectual development, there does appear to be an advantage to visual processing in these children. If so, then it may be helpful to teach elementary reading skills to children with Down syndrome. In short, until shown otherwise, Buckley et al.'s (1996) emphasis on reading instruction seems promising.

But when considering intellectual rates and profiles in Down syndrome, the most urgent need involves greater numbers of more detailed studies. Even though Down syndrome receives more behavioural studies than all other genetic disorders combined, we still know precious little about intellectual development in this syndrome. In essence, we need to take our preliminary findings about slowing intellectual development and visual-processing advantages, and work harder to discover why both occur, and what can be done to aid the intellectual development of children with Down syndrome.

References

Bernheimer LC, Keogh B (1988) Stability of cognitive performance of children with developmental delays. American Journal on Mental Retardation 92: 539-42.

Bernheimer LC, Keogh B, Guthrie D (1997) Stability and change over time in cognitive level of children with delays. American Journal on Mental Retardation 101: 365-73.

Buckley S, Bird G, Byrne A (1996) Practical and theoretical issues in literacy. In Rondal J, Nadel L, Perera J (eds) Down's Syndrome: Psychological, Psychobiological, and Socio-educational Perspectives. London: Whurr. pp. 119-28.

Carr J (1992) Longitudinal research in Down's syndrome. International Review of Research in Mental Retardation 18: 199-223.

Cunningham CC (1987) Early intervention in Down's syndrome. In Hoskins G, Murphy G (eds) Prevention of Mental Handicap: A World View. London: Royal Society of Medicine Services. pp. 169-82.

Dunst CJ (1988) Stage transitioning in the sensorimotor development of Down's syndrome infants. Journal of Mental Deficiency Research 32: 405-10.

Dykens EM (1995) Measuring behavioral phenotypes: Provocations from the 'New Genetics'. American Journal on Mental Retardation 99: 522-32.

Dykens EM, Hodapp RM, Evans DW (1994) Profiles and development of adaptive behavior in children with Down syndrome. American Journal on Mental Retardation 98: 580-7.

Fowler A (1990) The development of language structure in children with Down syndrome: Evidence for a specific syntactic delay. In Cicchetti D, Beeghly M (eds) Children with Down Syndrome: A Developmental Approach. New York: Cambridge University Press. pp. 302-28.

Gibson D (1966) Early developmental staging as a prophesy index in Down's Syndrome. American Journal of Mental Deficiency 70: 825-8.

Gibson D (1978) Down Syndrome: The Psychology of Mongolism. Cambridge: Cambridge University Press.

Hodapp RM (1996) Down syndrome: developmental, psychiatric, and management issues. Child and Adolescent Psychiatric Clinics of North America 5: 881-94.

Hodapp RM, Dykens EM (1994) Mental retardation's two cultures of behavioral research. American Journal on Mental Retardation 98: 675-87.

Hodapp RM, Leckman JF, Dykens EM, Sparrow SS, Zelinsky DG, Ort SI (1992) K-ABC profiles in children with fragile X syndrome, Down syndrome, and nonspecific mental retardation. American Journal on Mental Retardation 97: 39-46.

Hodapp RM, Zigler E (1990) Applying the developmental perspective to individuals with Down syndrome. In Cicchetti D, Beeghly M (eds) Children with Down Syndrome: A Developmental Perspective. New York: Cambridge University Press. pp. 1-28.

Marcell M, Armstrong V (1982) Auditory and visual sequential memory of Down syndrome and nonretarded children. American Journal of Mental Deficiency 87: 86-95.

McDade HL, Adler S (1980) Down syndrome and short-term memory impairment: A storage or retrieval deficit? American Journal of Mental Deficiency 84: 561-7.

Melyn M, White D (1973) Mental and developmental milestones of noninstitutionalized Down's syndrome children. Pediatrics 52: 542-5.

Miller JF (1992) Lexical development in young children with Down Syndrome. In Chapman R (ed) Processes in Language Acquisition and Disorders. St Louis: Mosby. pp. 202-16.

Morgan S (1979) Development and distribution of intellectual and adaptive skills in Down syndrome children: implications for early intervention. Mental Retardation 17: 247-9.

Pueschel S, Gallagher P, Zartler A, Pezzullo J (1987) Cognitive and learning processes in children with Down syndrome. Research in Developmental Disabilities 8: 21-37.

Silverstein AB (1982) A note on the constancy of IQ. American Journal of Mental Deficiency 87: 227-9.

Stavrou E (1990) The long-term stability of WISC-R scores in mildly retarded and learning disabled children. Psychology in the Schools 27: 101-10.

Chapter 12
Learning and Memory in Down Syndrome

LYNN NADEL

Introduction

Individuals with Down syndrome are mentally retarded, but just how, and how severely, remain unclear. The presumption of severe retardation meant that institutionalization was the norm through the 1950s and 60s, but this is now extremely rare. Instead, programmes of early stimulation are in use worldwide, with encouraging results. Only careful evaluation will show which forms of stimulation are most beneficial; but it is already clear that this generation is doing much better than those which preceded it.

This chapter will review what is known about one aspect of cognitive function in Down syndrome: learning and memory. It will start with discussion of current approaches to memory in normally developing individuals, to provide a context within which to understand the situation in Down syndrome. This discussion will include analysis of memory systems, their underlying neural bases, and how their emergence reflects neural maturation. Consideration of the cognitive and neural status of individuals with Down syndrome will follow. While we understand some aspects of the syndrome, much remains to be found out. Animal models of Down syndrome are beginning to prove very helpful in dissecting the cognitive deficits, and I will review some recent results in this area. The chapter will close with some discussion of the research needed in the future to bring greater understanding. Clear analysis of the pattern and diversity of deficits should permit the development of ever better forms of early stimulation, thereby ultimately fulfilling the goal of maximizing the potential of every child born with Down syndrome.

The Structure of Learning and Memory

In recent years it has become clear that learning and memory functions cannot be characterized in a singular fashion, either in terms of their behavioural and cognitive properties, or in terms of the neural systems upon which they rest. Initially in work with animals (eg, Nadel and O'Keefe 1974; O'Keefe and Nadel 1978), and subsequently in work with humans (eg, Cohen and Squire 1980), it has been shown that there are multiple learning and memory systems with distinct properties and neural bases. Understanding the nature of these multiple memory systems and their specific roles is relevant to the proper characterization of Down syndrome because the neural dysfunctions observed in this (and most other) syndromes are not spread evenly throughout the brain. Rather, they effect some parts of the brain more than others. To the extent that different brain regions are essential for quite different forms of learning and memory, it is critical to determine what kinds of learning and memory exist, what brain regions are responsible for each type, and what brain regions are particularly compromised in Down syndrome. Only when we have answers to these questions will we be able to state with some assurance just what aspects of learning and memory are especially at risk in this syndrome.

How Many Types of Learning and Memory Are There?

When the notion that there was more than one type of learning/memory first surfaced (eg, Gaffan 1974; Hirsh 1974; Nadel and O'Keefe 1974), it was common to think about two quite different types, with distinct behavioural properties and separate underlying neural substrates. Over the years researchers have proposed many different ways of characterizing these two systems, but certain common threads run through virtually all of these characterizations. Figure 12.1 presents a standard approach to this 'dual-system' analysis, separating memory into two broad types: *explicit* and *implicit*. This terminology was originally proposed by Schacter (1985), and has the virtue of being theoretically neutral in most respects, resting instead on operational characteristics. While these types of memory are quite difficult to define precisely in nonhuman experimental subjects, they are easier to apply in the human case, and hence appropriate for an analysis of Down syndrome.

Explicit memory is characterized by conscious recollection, and typically involves verbal recall. Examples of explicit memory include such things as episodes and events from one's life, facts about the world, and just about anything that one can talk about from the past. *Implicit memory*, by contrast, cannot be talked about, or brought to conscious awareness. Rather, it can merely be displayed through behaviour. Examples include motor skills such as learning to ride a bicycle or play squash, and cognitive skills such as learning to pronounce words in a foreign language or read mirror-reversed writing. Strong evidence that these two classes of memory are distinct comes from an analysis of individuals with various forms of amnesia. In most cases, explicit memory is profoundly impaired, but implicit memory remains largely within normal range.

Episodes, events and facts	Skills and habits

- yesterday's dinner
- Kennedy assassination
- capital of Spain is Madrid

- how to play tennis
- rules of chess

Explicit memory	Implicit memory

Figure 12.1 Two types of learning and memory.

In the past few years it has become obvious that this dichotomous approach is too simple, and that there are perhaps as many as five distinguishable forms of learning and memory. Figure 12.2 presents a five-way analysis that captures much of the current work in the field. It is important to discuss, at least briefly, current thinking about the neural substrates of these five kinds of learning/memory, because the facts of neural development in Down syndrome (as we see below) can best be understood by referring to these substrates. In what follows I briefly describe each type of learning.

1. *Sensory-perceptual features*: In this type of learning, information about the physical properties of things in the world is acquired. This includes learning how things look, sound, feel, taste and smell. It includes learning about how objects in the world behave with respect to motion, and gravity, such that one can respond appropriately to them (eg, get out of the way of a moving vehicle).
2. *Habits*: In this type of learning, behavioural skills are acquired, such that one can perform them in the future. This includes both motor skills (eg, hitting a golf ball), and cognitive skills (eg, solving a complex problem through iterative rules).
3. *Meaning*: In this type of learning, information about what things mean is acquired. The best example of this category is words, but also included is what we learn about the meaning and uses of objects.
4. *Value*: In this type of learning information about the valence of things and events is acquired. Examples include learning that chocolate tastes good, that quinine tastes bad, that touching fire hurts, and so on.
5. *Contexts*: This type of learning involves the acquisition of information about the spatial and temporal setting in which particular events transpired. Contextual information is essential to episode memory, the form of memory most impaired in amnesia.

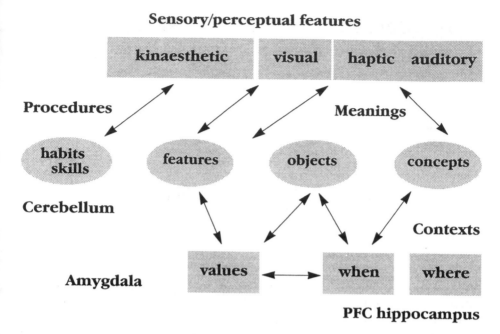

Figure 12.2 Five memory modules.

Brain Correlates of Memory Systems

Figure 12.3 indicates the brain structures currently thought to play an important role in each of these types of learning. The evidence for these assertions comes largely from three kinds of studies: those in which animals with lesions in structures of interest were tested on various kinds of learning; those in which neuronal recordings were made in animals performing various kinds of tasks; and those in which brain activation in humans was assessed with various neuroimaging techniques, such as positron emission tomography (PET), functional magnetic resonance imaging (fMRI), and event-related potential (ERP) recording. Such studies have shown that the sensory neocortex is critical for the ability to learn about the features of objects in the world (Gross et al. 1972); that the amygdala is essential for learning about the positive and negative aspects of things and events (LeDoux 1995); that certain frontal and temporal cortical structures influence the learning of words and the acquisition of semantic knowledge (eg, Martin et al. 1996); that the caudate nucleus and/or the cerebellum are involved in the acquisition of skills (Bizzi and Mussa-Ivaldi 1998); that the prefrontal cortex seems to be necessary for learning about the temporal aspects of experience (eg, Petrides 1994)); and that the hippocampal system is central to learning about space and spatial context (Nadel and Willner 1980; O'Keefe and Nadel 1978).

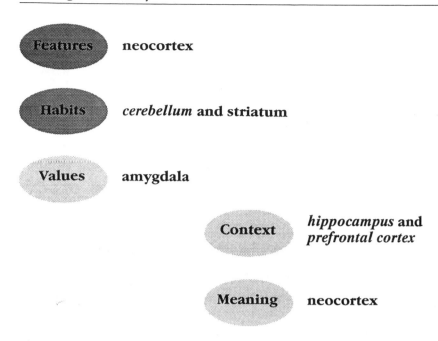

Figure 12.3 Brain systems thought to underlie the various forms of memory.

Development of Memory Systems

Not all these forms of learning are available to the newly born organism. The time at which each kind of learning emerges varies somewhat across species, making comparative analyses difficult. To compound matters, knowledge about the maturation of various brain structures in humans is still somewhat limited, in contrast to the wealth of data available on this issue in rodents and, to a lesser extent, primates.

Figure 12.4 presents, in an oversimplified way, current knowledge about the time of emergence of the various types of learning. Although matters are more complicated than this, the view that episodic memory emerges relatively late is quite well supported by available data.

These developmental facts are interesting in the context of the way in which learning and memory emerges in Down syndrome. Figure 12.5 provides an overview of the status of the different kinds of learning in individuals with Down syndrome. The figure shows that most, but not all, forms of implicit memory are preserved in Down syndrome, whereas many forms of explicit memory are impaired. A recent example of this pattern of neuropsychological deficits was provided by Carlesimo et al. (1997). They tested individuals with Down syndrome, mental-age matched control subjects, and subjects with non-Down syndrome mental retardation on a battery of tasks, allowing separate tests of implicit and explicit memory function. No deficit was observed in implicit memory (stem completion task), but deficits were observed in

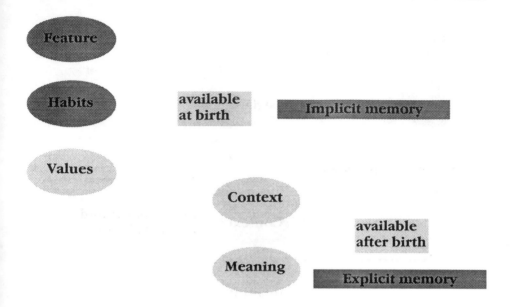

Figure 12.4 Development of the five forms of memory.

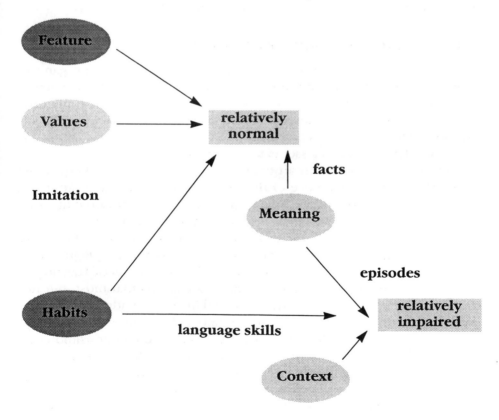

Figure 12.5 A summary of learning and memory capacities in Down syndrome.

explicit memory (word list learning, prose recall and figure reproduction). A survey of results from a number of studies (Table 12.1) is largely consistent with this conclusion. What is important to note in this table is the relatively normal profile shown by younger individuals with Down syndrome in a number of implicit memory tasks (operant and classical conditioning, imitation learning), and the deficits observed in explicit tasks (episodic memory).

This pattern is consistent with the suggestion that late-developing brain structures, and their functions, are particularly impaired in Down syndrome (Nadel 1986). In this regard, there is strong, but not incontrovertible, evidence that individuals with Down syndrome perform particularly poorly on tasks requiring the hippocampus, prefrontal cortex and, perhaps, cerebellum.

Table 12.2 presents the volumes of various brain areas in controls and in individuals with Down syndrome. The overall decrease in brain volume of about 30 per cent reflects considerable heterogeneity from one brain area to the next. A handful of areas show decreases that are considerably smaller, and these structures are typically closer to the sensory or motor side (eg, precentral and postcentral gyri, caudate). More central structures, which do indeed mature later, show the larger decreases (eg, prefrontal cortex, hippocampus, cerebellum). There are two anomalous findings that suggest the need for more data (a very substantial decrease in the anterior cingulate, and a paradoxical increase in the parahippocampal gyrus).

Animal Models of Down Syndrome

Much can be gained by the study of animal model systems that capture some aspect of Down syndrome. In the past 10-15 years increasingly refined genetic techniques have permitted the creation of progressively more realistic mouse models. The initial model (trisomy 16) was of limited use because these animals were not viable past birth. More recently, partially trisomic mice have been created that express triplication for those parts of chromosome 16 most closely related to the critical band on human chromosome 21 known to be responsible for much of the phenotype of Down syndrome. One model in particular has been studied quite extensively, the Ts65Dn mouse (Davisson and Costa, in press).

The behavioural work with this mouse is quite compelling - selective deficits have been observed in behavioural situations requiring the hippocampus (exploration and spatial learning, Coussons-Read and Crnic 1996, Escorihuela et al. 1995; maze learning, Reeves et al. 1995). Going beyond the behavioural domain, a number of studies have now shown specific neurobiological defects in hippocampal function in the Ts65Dn mouse. Siarey et al. (1997), for example, have shown that hippocampal synaptic plasticity (LTP) is reduced in these mice, and Dierssen et al. (1996) reported impairments in metabolic processes in the hippocampus of these mice that could be related to the deficits in plasticity.

Table 12.1 Learning and memory

Habituation	foetus	abnormal
Operant conditioning	3 months	normal
Contingency learning	9 months	impaired
Object concept development	4–33 months	unstable
Imitation learning	55 months	normal
Counting principles	9.7 years	normal
Orienting response	9.8 years	normal
Episodic memory	23 years	impaired
Word learning	23 years	normal
Classical conditioning	27.6 years	normal
Classical conditioning	47.7 years	impaired
Object/location learning	33.6 years	impaired

Table 12.2 Volumes of various brain areas in controls and in individuals with Down syndrome

Structure	Controls	Down syndrome	% change
Cerebrum	1101.26 ± 144.49	784.01 ± 20.46	−28.8
Prefrontal cortex	40.27 ± 9.03	30.17 ± 3.78	−25.1
Ant. cingulate	2.68 ± 0.74	0.72 ± 0.33	−73.1
Inf. parietal	8.95 ± 1.90	6.49 ± 1.24	−27.5
Precentral gyrus	5.30 ± 0.73	4.80 ± 0.62	−9.4
Inf. temporal	11.32 ± 1.85	9.11 ± 0.90	−19.5
Postcentral gyrus	8.68 ± 1.70	7.33 ± 0.50	−15.5
Hippocampus	5.80 ± 0.74	4.28 ± 0.35	−26.2
Caudate	7.39 ± 1.18	6.28 ± 0.80	−15.0
Cerebellum	119.90 ± 13.10	84.37 ± 5.07	−29.6
Parahippocamp.	5.98 ± 1.09	6.96 ± 0.99	+16.4

Source: Raz et al. 1995

More recently, another partially trisomic mouse has been studied, the Ts108Cje variant (Sage et al. 1996). This mouse is trisomic for only a portion of the region triplicated in the Ts65Dn mouse, hence its study should permit a finer analysis of the relation between specific genes and particular features of the Down syndrome phenotype.

Conclusions and Implications

Research on individuals with Down syndrome and in animal models has provided an increasingly detailed sense of which aspects of learning and memory are relatively preserved and which are disproportionately impaired. The data strongly support the view that implicit memory functions are generally unimpaired, while explicit memory functions are deficient. This pattern is consistent with data from a variety of neurobiological studies indicating that a particular subset of brain regions is most seriously affected in this syndrome - the hippocampus, the prefrontal cortex and perhaps the cerebellum. In the coming years careful neuropsychological study of individuals with Down syndrome should concentrate on clarifying this pattern, by using tasks that are known to require these neural structures. In combination with the use of ever more precise animal models, we can expect that this research will, in the course of the next decade, provide a much clearer picture of why mental retardation results from trisomy 21. With this kind of knowledge in hand, it should be possible to plan intervention strategies that will result in ever better prognoses for individuals with Down syndrome. This vision of the future provides reason for great hope, even as it indicates the significant challenge that remains before us.

References

Bizzi E, Mussa-Ivaldi FA (1998) Neural basis of motor control and its cognitive implications. Trends in Cognitive Sciences 2: 97-102.

Carlesimo GA, Marotta L, Vicari S (1997) Long-term memory in mental retardation: Evidence for a specific impairment in subjects with Down's syndrome. Neuropsychologia 35: 71-9.

Cohen NJ, Squire L (1980) Preserved learning and retention of pattern-analyzing skill in amnesia: dissociation of 'knowing how' and 'knowing that'. Science 210: 207-9.

Coussons-Read ME, Crnic LS (1996) Behavioral assessment of the Ts65Dn mouse, a model for Down syndrome: altered behavior in the elevated plus maze and open field. Behavior Genetics 26: 7-13.

Davisson MT, Costa AC (in press) Mouse models of Down syndrome.

Dierssen M, Vallina IF, Baamonde C, Lumbreras MA, Martinez-Cue C, Calatayid SG, Florez J (1996) Impaired cyclic AMP production in the hippocampus of a Down syndrome murine model. Developmental Brain Research 95: 122-4.

Escorihuela RM, Fernandez-Teruel A, Vallina IF, Baamjonde C, Lumbreras MA, Dierssen M, Tobena A, Florez J (1995) A behavioral assessment of Ts65Dn mice: a putative Down syndrome model. Neuroscience Letters 199: 143-6.

Gaffan D (1974) Recognition impaired and association intact in the memory of monkeys after transection of the fornix. Journal of Comparative and Physiological Psychology 86: 1100-9.

Gross CJ, Roche-Muranda CE, Bender DB (1972) Visual properties of neurons in inferotemporal cortex of the macaque. Journal of Neurophysiology 35: 96-111.

Hirsh R (1974) The hippocampus and contextual retrieval from memory: a theory. Behavioral Biology 12: 421-44.

LeDoux JD (1995) Emotion: clues from the brain. Annual Review of Psychology 46: 209-35.

Martin A, Wiggs CL, Ungerleider LG, Haxby JV (1996) Neural correlates of category-specific knowledge. Nature 379: 649-52.

Nadel L (1986) Down syndrome in neurobiological perspective. In Epstein CJ (ed) The Neurobiology of Down syndrome. New York: Raven Press. pp. 239-51.

Nadel L, O'Keefe J (1974) The hippocampus in pieces and patches: an essay on modes of explanation in physiological psychology. In Bellairs R, Gray EG (eds) Essays on the Nervous System. A Festschrift for JZ Young. Oxford: The Clarendon Press.

Nadel L, Willner J (1980) Context and conditioning: a place for space. Physiological Psychology 8: 218-28.

O'Keefe J, Nadel L (1978) The Hippocampus as a Cognitive Map. Oxford: The Clarendon Press.

Petrides M (1994) Frontal lobes and working memory: evidence from investigations of the effects of cortical excisions in nonhuman primates. In Boller F, Grafman J (eds) Handbook of Neuropsychology, Vol. 9. Amsterdam: Elsevier. pp. 59-82.

Raz N, Torres IJ, Briggs SD, Spencer WD, Thornton AE, Loken, WJ, Gunning FM, McQuain JD, Drisen NR, Acker JD (1995) Selective neuroanatomic abnormalities in Down's syndrome and their cognitive correlates. Neurology, 45: 356-66.

Reeves RH, Irving NG, Moran TH, Wohn A, Kitt C, Sisodia SS, Schnidt C, Bronson RT, Davisson MT (1995) A mouse model for Down syndrome exhibits learning and behaviour deficits. Nature Genetics 11: 177-84.

Sage H, Huang TT, Carlson EJ, Epstein CJ (1996) A new partial trisomy of murine chromosome 16 (Ts108Cje) as an animal model for Down syndrome. American Journal of Human Genetics 59 (supplement): A22.

Schacter DL (1985) Multiple forms of memory in humans and animals. In Weinberger NM, McGaugh JL, Lynch G (eds) Memory Systems of the Brain. New York: The Guilford Press. pp. 351-79.

Siarey RJ, Stoll J, Rapoport SI, Galdzicki Z (1997) Altered long-term potentiation in the young and old Ts65Dn mouse, a model for Down syndrome. Neuropharmacology 36: 1549-54.

Chapter 13
Language in Down Syndrome: Current Perspectives

JEAN A RONDAL

As a result of more than 25 years of extensive research efforts, the nature and the extent of the language problems in persons with Down syndrome have become better known. Table 13.1 summarizes the major data in this respect (for a full review and discussion, see Rondal and Edwards 1997).

It is important to stress the normalcy principle, ie, the fundamental normality of language development in Down syndrome, because this question has been at the centre of technical discussion for quite some time. The empirical indications now available point in the same direction, ie, *language development in Down syndrome follows the same sequences and establishes the same dedicated mind structures* in Down syndrome as in nonretarded people. What differs is that Down syndrome language development is slower and often remains incomplete. Basically, however, development is the same as in nonretarded people. For a corresponding developmental or delay point of view on Down syndrome regarding nonlanguage areas, see, for example, the work of Cicchetti (eg, Cicchetti and Beeghly 1990).

Given the indications in Table 13.1, can one speak of *specific* language problems in Down syndrome? Strictly speaking, 'specific' means that some or all language difficulties in Down syndrome are *pathognomonic*, ie, denoting one or more typical symptoms for the condition and *not found in any other condition* (*Stedman's Medical Dictionary* 1990). This is clearly not the case for the language problems associated with Down syndrome. Each one of these problems can be found (to different extents, however) in other mental retardation syndromes, genetic or otherwise. More generally, it can be proposed that there is no diagnostic linguistic or behavioural *single feature* that would independently separate persons with various mental retardation syndromes (eg, Down syndrome, Williams' syndrome, Fragile-X syndrome, Cri-du-Chat syndrome, Trisomy 18, Trisomy 13, and so on).

Table 13.1 Major language problems in persons with Down syndrome

Language component	Semiology
1. Sound articulation and auditory discrimination	* *Articulatory and co-articulatory difficulties, particularly with the more delicate phonemes.* – Slow and sometimes incomplete maturation of phonemic discrimination.
2. Lexical semantics	– Reduced lexicon both in number of lexemes and in semantic features within lexemes. * *Poor organization of the mental lexicon, both semantically and pregrammatically.*
3. Morpho-syntax	– Reduced length and formal complexity of utterances. * *Problems with inflexional morphology.* – Problems with producing and understanding subordinated propositions and compound sentences.
4. Language pragmatics	– Slowness of development in the advanced pragmatic skills (eg, topic contribution in conversation, interpersonal requests, monitoring verbal interactions with other people).
5. Discursive organisation	* *Insufficiently developed discourse macrostructures.*

* The asterisks signal the most recurrent and difficult problems for efficient language intervention. See Rondal and Edwards (1997) for a full analysis.

Specificity is found (see Rondal 1995a; Rondal and Edwards 1997), not at the level of the separate symptoms but at a more systemic (syndromic) level of analysis. In many (perhaps most) mental retardation syndromes (particularly the genetic ones), there exists a particular set of language characteristics justifying the specificity claim. This claim is illustrated below with data relative to Down syndrome, Williams' syndrome, and affected males with Fragile-X syndrome (Table 13.2).

As shown in Table 13.2, the language profiles of Down syndrome, Williams' syndrome, and affected male Fragile-X syndrome subjects differ in ways that are not related to the psychometric levels in each syndrome. Additional research is needed to analyse these comparisons in more detail and to extend the syndromic profile search to a larger number of mental retardation aetiological categories.

One reasonable possibility is that the semiological differences between mental retardation entities correspond to syndrome differences in brain anatomy and physiology. Research is being conducted in several places to unravel these substrate variations. They will help to specify the brain organization of various syndromes conducive to mental retardation.

The syndrome-specific indications also supply interesting pieces of evidence that should be used in clinical work to constrain remediation programmes. Patterns of development in a mentally retarded individual may be, at least partly, aetiology-specific. Professionals should try as far as possible to tailor their interventions to specific aetiological groups. Intervention programmes will work better when the child's aetiology is among several important characteristics (eg, individual differences, age-related issues, language modularity) considered in designing language remediation. This objective can be fully met when more data have been gathered on a larger number of mental retardation syndromes.

Table 13.2 Three MR syndromic profiles for speech and language

Language aspect	Down's	Syndromes Williams	Fragile-X (affected males)
Phonetico-phonological	– –	+	– –
Lexical	–	+ +	+
Thematic semantic	+	+	?
Morpho-syntactic	– –	+ (comprehension?)	–
Pragmatic	+	– –	–
Discursive	– –	+	–

Key: +(+): relative strength; –(–): relative weakness; ?: insufficient data available. See Rondal and Edwards 1997.

It is also of primary importance to stress the interindividual differences existing in virtually all aspects of language among individuals with Down syndrome. The final levels of development reached by Down syndrome persons in language cannot be predicted with certainty from the beginning (this is also the case for nonretarded individuals). The implication is that one should provide each Down syndrome infant, child, and adolescent with optimal language stimulation and training in the hope that he/she will reach advanced levels of language functioning, or at least that the best possible level for each individual will be reached at the end of development.

It is quite possible, and indeed likely, that individual language abilities in the Down syndrome population (as well as other abilities, such as cognitive ones) are distributed according to a Gaussian curve. This means that for every language component one may expect that a majority of Down syndrome persons will score in the central part of the Down syndrome distribution while a few score at the two extremes of the same distribution. The latter cases are either exceptionally favoured or exceptionally restricted as to the final levels reached in development. I have reported elsewhere (see Rondal 1995b, 1998) on exceptional cases of language development in Down syndrome, and particularly on the astonishing case of one Down syndrome adult woman presenting normal to quasinormal productive and receptive functioning in the formal aspects of language; these very aspects usually prove most difficult for Down syndrome persons.

I have suggested (Rondal 1998) that the phenotypic distribution of language abilities in Down syndrome persons, including the exceptional cases, could correspond to interindividual differences in the dedicated brain architectures; these brain differences themselves are probably related to (and presumably caused by) genotypic variations at the level of chromosome 21. We go then from variations at the level of the genes to variations at the level of dedicated brain centres for language to variations in behavioural language ability.

Results of neuropathological studies of the brain of Down syndrome persons reveal major anomalies, including arrested maturation of neurons and synapses some time around birth, reduced brain weight, reduced neuronal densities, decreased synaptic density and presynaptic length, hypoplasia of the frontal lobes, narrowed superior temporal gyri, delayed myelination of nerve fibres affecting long associative and intercortical fibres between frontal and temporal lobes, hypothalamic and hippocampal abnormalities, and diminished size of brain stem and cerebellum (Nadel 1996; Wisnieswky et al. 1996). One brain region particularly affected, in addition to the temporal cortex, is the inferior frontal gyrus including Broca's area, as indicated by recent PET scan studies of cerebral metabolic patterns in young Down syndrome adults (eg, Horowitz et al. 1990).

It is reasonable to assume that the brain problems of Down syndrome individuals undermine the development and functioning of their language structures. Most likely to be particularly detrimental is the reported slowing down of synaptic growth around birth (Nadel 1996). The consequence is that Down syndrome subjects often do not possess the necessary brain architecture for fully accommodating language stimuli in such a way as to spontaneously construct full grammatical knowledge. The language-exceptional Down syndrome subjects escape the above fate for reasons that may be related to the phenotypic effects of genetic variation. The same suggestion is valid for other genetic syndromes as well. Geneticists agree that there is substantial variation at the genetic level between people *within* genotypic categories such as Down syndrome, Williams' syndrome, Fragile-X syndrome, and other genetic causes of mental retardation (Dykens 1995). Korenberg et al. (1994) constructed a phenotypic map including 25 features considered typical of Down syndrome. They assign a region of 2-20 megabases between regions p11.2 and 22.3 on the distal part of the long arm of chromosome 21, as likely to contain the genes responsible for the Down syndrome phenotypes. This conception of the genotype-phenotype relationship in Down syndrome is consistent with central characteristics of T21, such as the rich variety of phenotypes and the variability in both penetrance (ie, the proportion of individuals with the susceptible genes having the disorder) and expression of the Down syndrome features. It is conceivable that important interindividual variation existing at the level of brain architecture in the language areas of Down syndrome persons results from genetic differences and that these variations probably cause individual differences in formal abilities.

The brain-genes perspective defined above has the advantage of proposing one single explanatory perspective for the range of variation observed in the language of typical mental retardation/Down syndrome people and the extremes of such variation in the language-exceptional cases. It may also be applied to behavioural and brain differences across genetic syndromes such as Down syndrome, Williams' syndrome, and Fragile-X syndrome; a large number of other genetic syndromes awaiting systematic phenotypical studies (Dykens1995).

Turning to the educational level, the good news is that at last identifiable progress is being made in language remediation with Down syndrome children. Significant advances on previous timetables for several important aspects of language development in Down syndrome are currently recorded by practicians, if not precisely measured and published. This means that we are developing the technology for markedly reducing some of the most usual delays in the language development of Down syndrome persons. Language acquisition is a cumulative process. This implies that important gains early in development will have positive consequences for subsequent acquisitions and are likely to allow the child to proceed further in his/her development than would have been the case otherwise.

From current remedial experience, it seems that at least one or two developmental years, sometimes more, can be gained early in language development by relying on particular techniques. For example, systematic prelinguistic training followed in the second year of life by a systematic combination of gestural signs and words will markedly favour lexical and early combinatorial acquisitions in most Down syndrome children. It shortens the period of time between prelinguistic functioning and early language in Down syndrome, a period that in the past could extend over two or even three years, to the desperation of many parents.

Later on (ie, around two or three years chronological age), it may be useful to train both written and oral language at the same time, using appropriate methods. Among other benefits, this is proving to be an efficient way of promoting morpho-syntactic regulations in Down syndrome, in exploiting the better preserved visuo-spatial channel in these children, to help the more feeble auditory-vocal one.

Research findings also indicate that adequate schooling and care of Down syndrome persons have the consequence of improving achievement levels in language abilities. As noted by Rynders (this book), for example, these developments place many Down syndrome students at a level of literacy and personal abilities sufficient for meeting the functional demands of everyday community life, with some Down syndrome individuals achieving considerably beyond these average levels.

Not enough parents and professionals (psychologists, physicians, educators, and so on) have sufficient knowledge of these new findings and the interesting perspectives they open. Old stereotypes of Down syndrome infants, children, adolescents, and adults as incapacitated and poorly functioning people still prevail in too many places. Sometimes, even today, some paediatricians, child psychologists, or speech therapists warn desperate parents that a large number of Down syndrome individuals fail to develop language to any significant extent. This of course is utterly false. It is clear now that the vast majority of Down syndrome children, when properly cared for and trained, will learn to speak, to express themselves verbally, and to use functionally adequate - if not always formally perfect - language. This renders them able to become responsible and productive citizens and, when offered the opportunity, to develop in remarkable ways.

Here we have two related problems that need to be better dealt with in the coming years. First, we need to *inform* various communities better about the real potential of Down syndrome persons. Second, we need to *train* better professionals in the fields related to Down syndrome (as well as to other mental retardation syndromes) in order to make them increasingly able to translate more rapidly and efficiently the applicable research knowledge into practical field realities.

References

Cicchetti D, Beeghly M (eds) (1990) Children with Down Syndrome: A Developmental Perspective. New York: Cambridge University Press.

Dykens E (1995) Measuring behavioral phenotypes: provocations from the 'new genetics'. American Journal on Mental Retardation 99: 522-32.

Horowitz B, Schapiro M, Grady C, Rapaport S (1990) Cerebral metabolic pattern in young adult Down's syndrome subjects: altered intercorrelations between regional rates of glucose utilisation. Journal of Mental Deficiency Research 34: 237-52.

Korenberg JR, Chen X-N, Schipper R, Sun Z, Gonsky R, Gerwehr S, Carpenter N, Daumer C, Dignan P, Disteche C, Graham JM, Hugdins Jr I, McGillivray B, Miyazaki K, Ogasawara N, Park JP, Pagon R, Pueschel S, Sack G, Say B, Schuffenhauer S, Soukup S, Yamanaka T (1994) Down syndrome phenotype: the consequence of chromosomal imbalance. Proceedings of the National Academy of Sciences of the USA, 91: 4997-5001.

Nadel L (1996) Learning, memory and neural function in Down's syndrome. In Rondal JA, Perera J, Nadel L, Comblain A (eds) Down's Syndrome: Psychological, Psychobiological and Socio-educational Perspectives. London: Whurr. pp. 21-42.

Rondal JA (1995a). Especificidad sistemica del lenguaje en el síndrome de Down. In Perera J (Ed) Especificidad en el Síndrome de Down. Barcelona: Masson. pp. 91-107.

Rondal JA (1995b) Exceptional Language Development in Down Syndrome. Implications for the Cognition-Language Relationship. New York: Cambridge University Press.

Rondal JA (1998) Cases of exceptional language in mental retardation and Down syndrome: Explanatory perspectives. Down Syndrome 5: 1-15.

Rondal JA, Edwards S (1997). Language in Mental Retardation. London: Whurr.

Stedman's Medical Dictionary (1990) Baltimore, MD: Williams and Wilkins.

Wisniewski K, Kida E, Brown W (1996) Consequences of genetic abnormalities in Down's syndrome on brain structure and function. In Rondal JA, Perera J, Nadel L, Comblain A (eds) Down's Syndrome: Psychological, Psychobiological and Socio-educational Perspectives. London: Whurr. pp. 3-39.

PART 5
MEDICINE

Chapter 14
The Present State of Medical Knowledge in Down Syndrome

ALBERTO RASORE-QUARTINO

Down syndrome is a major cause of mental retardation, associated with distinctive facial and physical features, congenital anomalies of the heart and of the gastrointestinal tract; it carries an increased risk of leukemia, defects of the immune system and of Alzheimer disease. Its prevalence is about 1/1,000 at birth and decreases regularly thereafter (Epstein 1995). In recent years better health care and decreased recourse to placement in institutions have had beneficial effects on the life of these persons, both in length and quality. Life expectancy is consequently greatly increased, changing from 9 years in 1929, to 12 years in 1947, to 52 years in 1970 and showing the same trend in the last decade (Baird and Sadovnick 1988). For the future we can foresee a reduction in the birth of babies with Down syndrome, due both to the general reduction of birth rate and to the effects of largely diffused prenatal diagnosis. In combination with the prolonged survival rate, we can expect in a given population a decreasing number of children and a relative increase of adults and aged persons with Down syndrome. This will certainly change our attitude and strategies towards the syndrome.

A fundamental clue to the explication of complex phenotype determination in DS is the consequence of present studies showing specific effects of increased dosage of genes on chromosome 21. Clinical observations made it possible to conclude that a small region of chromosome 21, band 22 of the long arm, contains a cluster of genes that may independently contribute to the development of the brain, heart, gastrointestinal tract and immune system. This cluster of genes may also contribute to the genesis of some dysmorphic features, such as epicantal folds, Brushfield spots and other phenotypic marks (Korenberg et al. 1990).

Although relatively few genes are known that are located on chromosome 21, nevertheless it is tempting to speculate on the relationships existing between any single gene and a specific phenotype. So, abnormalities in the expression of the major structural protein of the ocular lens

153

(CRYA 1) may predispose to cataract; it is possible that interferon receptors (IFNA/BR) are related to immune defects and that the oncogene ETS2 is related to leukemia or to developmental defects.; overexpression of the Amyloid-beta-Precursor-Protein (APP) gene may be responsible for the early deposition of amyloid beta/A4 protein in the neuritic plaques of the brain, thus beginning the process leading to Alzheimer disease. Superoxide dismutase (SOD) is generally considered a protective enzyme, since it catalizes the transformation of superoxide radicals to hydrogen peroxide, which in turn is metabolized to water by glutathion peroxidase and catalase. But hydrogen peroxide is itself toxic and may give rise to more dangerous hydroxyl radicals in combination with superoxide. Increased SOD activity then can have effects on oxygen metabolytes and this could have deleterious consequences (Korenberg et al. 1994).

Congenital heart disease is the most common malformation. About 50 per cent of newborns are affected, representing 7 per cent of all children with congenital heart defects. Endocardial cushion defect (ECD), or atrioventricular canal defect, is the prevailing anomaly, averaging nearly half of the total (36-47%): it is followed by ventricular septal defect (26-33%), by patent ductus arteriosus (8-10%) and, to a lesser extent, by atrial septal defect and Tetralogy of Fallot (Tubman et al. 1992). In humans, ECD occurs either in isolated form or as a part of a malformation syndrome. Down syndrome and Ivermark syndrome (situs ambiguus with splenic anomalies) are most often associated with ECD. Isolated forms are more commonly associated with other cardiovascular malformations than syndromic forms. The complete form of ECD is also significantly more frequent in Down syndrome and in an animal model, mouse trisomy 16. All these facts suggest that specific genetic factors inherent in the trisomy are involved in the morphogenesis of ECD. Associated noncardiac anomalies have a similar pattern and frequency both with and without ECD. Moreover, the systems involved are mostly of the gastrointestinal or genitourinary tracts. It has been proposed that these tissues might constitute an embryological developmental field that is affected as a unit by the action of heterogeneous dysmorphic forces. It can be provisionally concluded that the overall cardiovascular 'phenotype' in syndromic ECD (ie, Down syndrome) is the net result of an interaction between syndromic determinants and the ECD process (Carmi et al. 1992). An early diagnosis of the congenital heart defects is desirable (echocardiography at birth), since most of them are treatable by effective surgery. Cardiac anomalies with increased pulmonary flow are very frequent. Affected children become symptomatic at an early age, developing pulmonary artery hypertension, cardiomegaly, cirrhosis of the liver and severe congestive heart failure. Patients show growth impairment and recurrent respiratory infections, resulting in high morbidity and mortality. Pulmonary vascular obstructive disease is a severe complication, the development of which generally prevents surgical correction (Spicer 1984).

Less data is available on cardiac status of adults with Down syndrome, compared with children. The recent literature shows that they can have cardiac problems other than congenital defects. The most frequent anomalies found in asymptomatic adults are mitral valve prolapse (MVP) and aortic regurgitation (AR), with a prevalence up to 70 per cent. These defects seem to occur only in adults, since they have never been detected in childhood (Goldhaber et al. 1987). MVP has been associated with disorders characterized by laxity of connective tissue, such as Marfan's or Ehlers-Danlos syndromes. In the same way, the connective tissue abnormalities present in Down syndrome might explain the increased frequency of these cardiac defects. Obviously, accurate diagnostic investigations are recommended in young adults, especially before dental and surgical procedures, for the detection of valve defects. Antibiotic prophylaxis for endocarditis should also be taken into consideration.

Other congenital malformations, although quite uncommon, are more frequent than in normal infants. Among gastrointestinal anomalies, duodenal stenosis, found in 4-7 per cent of newborns with Down syndrome, represents 30-50 per cent of all duodenal stenoses. Hirschprung's disease is found in 3-4 per cent of infants with Down syndrome, versus 0.02 per cent in other infants. Pancreas annulare and anal imperforation are also relatively frequent.

Linear growth retardation is a characteristic of Down syndrome. Stature is generally stabilized at minus 2-3 standard deviations on normal growth charts. The mechanisms responsible for short stature are not yet completely explained. A great deal of interest has focused on the role of somatomedins/insulin like growth factors (IGF), as these peptides are not only essential for body growth, but also for the development and maintenance of the nervous system. In a recent study, we showed that in children with Down syndrome, IGF-I is low or clearly pathological, with values similar to those found in hypopituitarism. Defective GH secretion has been hypothesized as a cause of short stature in Down syndrome (Castells et al. 1992). However, decreased IGF concentration does not seem to be accompanied by impaired GH responsiveness to secretogogues (Barreca et al. 1994). Most authors have confirmed normal GH secretion. Our results appear to exclude the notion that short stature and reduced IGF-I concentrations in Down syndrome are due to an alteration of GH secretion or of the GH receptor and point out the occurrence of a GH molecular anomaly in some of these patients (Barreca et al. 1994). GH treatment has been proposed in children with Down syndrome and impaired growth, irrespective of GH and IGF-I levels. Interesting results have been obtained, with acceleration of growth velocity (Anneren et al. 1993). Nevertheless, at present, the role of that therapy is still controversial, given the lack of long-term experience, the possibility of complications (hypertension, hyperglycaemia) and the risk of leukemia.

Sensory defects, when present, have considerable importance in the general pattern of mental development of children with Down syndrome, since they can significantly reduce the efficacy of any rehabilitation programme, even the most promising one. This is particularly true in the first years of life. Ocular abnormalities are definitely more common than in other children. From a practical point of view, it is necessary to point out the clinical significance of strabismus and of refractory defects, that can hinder correct vision and hence add an organic defect to the underlying mental impairment. An early diagnosis is warranted in order to correct these defects as early as possible. Surgical correction should also be provided, if necessary. It is well known that even very young children do not have difficulty in wearing spectacles if they receive real benefits. Cataract is another excessively frequent ocular defect observed both in newborns and adults.

When children with Down syndrome have some sort of hearing abnormality, they cannot employ the complex strategies necessary to compensate for their cognitive deficiencies. Conflicting data on the frequency of hearing abnormalities have been reported. Evidence suggests an excess of middle-ear pathology. A characteristic serous otitis can develop in the first years of life and often persists through adulthood. In fact, all the proposed treatments for ear infections, either medical or surgical, have a low success rate and hearing problems are the consequence of delayed recovery. From 75 to 80 per cent of persons with Down syndrome have a more or less severe hearing deficit, mostly a conductive one. It seems therefore of the utmost importance to adopt a preventive approach to the hearing problems of children with DS, in order to help them keep good communication abilities and satisfying socialization.

Immune function in Down syndrome has been investigated extensively, based on the well-known high incidence of infections and malignancies. Respiratory diseases and other infectious disorders are still a major cause of mortality, even if advances in chemotherapy and general health care have largely reduced the mortality rate. The assumption that Down syndrome is associated with an abnormal immune response was ultimately confirmed by many authors, although controversial results have been obtained (Ugazio et al. 1990). Both cell-mediated immunity and antibody-mediated immunity show complex anomalies. The thymus itself is smaller than in normal subjects of the same age. A marked thymocyte depletion, poor corticomedullary demarcation and a thin cortex are a universal finding. Hassal corpuscles are larger and their number increased. Defective production of thymic humoral factors has been reported by some authors, some of whom paralleled the reduction of thymic hormone with that occurring in normal ageing persons (Fabris et al. 1984). The number of T-lymphocytes expressing CD3 and CD4 antigens can be reduced, while circulating CD8 positive lymphocytes are either normal or increased; so are the cells with an NK phenotype. As for antibody-mediated immunity, conflicting data have been reported, depending mainly on the age of the population studied. In general, IgG and IgA serum levels are normal or increased, while that of IgM is normal or reduced. Although an increase of respiratory infections has been observed in children with Down syndrome, we recently inferred that bronchial asthma is, on the contrary, significantly lower (Forni et al. 1990), suggesting that the immunodeficiency state in Down syndrome may confer some protection against its development.

Persons with Down syndrome have a high frequency of autoantibodies and also an increased occurrence of autoimmune disorders, such as thyroid disorders, chronic active hepatitis, alopecia areata, thrombocytopenia. Autoimmunity may reflect an unbalanced immune control in Down syndrome, probably conditioned by defective T-cell control mechanisms. Production of some important cytokines is depressed and the phagocytes show functional impairment, exhibiting low chemotactic ability and reduced production of oxygen radicals.

In trisomic newborns, inefficient regulation of myelopoiesis is usual, its cause being either delayed maturation or a deficiency of committed stem cells (Weinstein 1978). Generalized cellular dysfunction is substantiated by the presence of various haematological abnormalities: polycytemia, thrombocytopenia, thrombocytosis, higher or lower leukocyte count. These abnormalities are time-limited and are the consequence of defective control in the production of haemopoietic cells in one or more cell lines (Miller and Cosgriff 1983). The extreme aspect of defective hemopoiesis is leukemia. In Down syndrome the risk of developing leukemia is 10 to 20 times higher than in normal children (Rosner and Lee 1972). The ratio Acute Lymphocytic Leukemia/Acute non Lymphocytic Leukemia is similar in both populations, except for the first two years of life. The response to the treatment, prognosis and other characteristics is similar. The abnormal sensitivity to methotrexate found in children with Down syndrome correlates with the prolonged clearance of the drug in these persons (Garrè et al. 1987). In Down syndrome 25 per cent of all leukemias are evident at birth; 15 per cent of the congenital leukemias develop in newborns with Down syndrome. In 17 per cent of Down syndrome infants, moreover, a form of acute, transitory leukemia, mainly of the myeloid type, can develop. Its clinical and haematological features are undistinguishable from those of common acute leukemia, except for the spontaneous and complete remission. Differential diagnosis is usually very difficult and severe problems can arise for therapeutic decisions (Cominetti et al 1985). Acute transitory leukemia would represent a myelodysplastic prephase of megakaryoblastic leukemia, with thrombocytopenia, lasting from several months to a few years. In Down syndrome megakaryoblastic leukemia has a 500-fold higher than expected incidence, with its peak under four years of age (Creutzig et al. 1996).

Since the first descriptions of Down syndrome and for almost a century, hypothyroidism was considered a constant feature of the syndrome. Only when laboratory tests for thyroid function became available did evidence spring up that most persons with Down syndrome are actually euthyroid. Nevertheless, it was also demonstrated that a higher incidence of thyroid disorders, chiefly hypothyroidism, is characteristic of Down syndrome. According to the literature, congenital hypothyroidism in Down syndrome varies from 0.7 per cent to 10 per cent, while in nontrisomic newborns it varies from 0.015 per cent to 0.020 per cent. Figures for acquired hypothyroidism are also largely variable (from 13% to 54% in Down syndrome, versus 0.8% to 1.1% in the normal population; Fort et al. 1984). Two forms of hypothyroidism can be distinguished, the most frequent one, the so-called compensated hypothyroidism, involves increased TSH levels, while T3 and T4 levels are within normal limits: it can be assumed to be a temporary phase preceding a probable hypofunctional condition. Increased TSH represents a central response to the reduction of functional thyroid tissue, on an immunological basis, and is followed by a progressive decrease of T3 and T4 values. Although this is commonly the course of the disease, in Down syndrome TSH levels often fluctuate without any modification of thyroid function. These transient thyroid neuroregulatory dysfunctions are possibly related to inappropriate secretion of TSH or to reduced sensitivity to TSH itself. An increased frequency of antithyroid antibodies is also found. Some authors found significantly lower IQs in persons with Down syndrome and elevated TSH.

Generally, hypothyroidism in Down syndrome is the consequence of an autoimmune disorder. Initially, only increased TSH values are detected, then the hormone deficiency develops, showing reduced T3 and T4 dosage. As the disease progresses, clinical symptoms appear. Unfortunately, they may not be recognized or can be mistaken for the features of the syndrome itself (dullness, increased fatigability, loss of attention and so on) mainly in adolescents and adults. Periodic tests of thyroid function are therefore mandatory. Since untreated hypothyroidism can interfere with normal neuronal function, causing decreased intellectual abilities, appropriate substitutive therapy is strongly recommended. The results of our investigations confirm that persons with Down syndrome are at increased risk of developing hypothyroidism at any age (Rasore-Quartino and Cominetti 1994). One person out of 12 has either compensated or subclinical hypothyroidism. Only recently has the relationship between Down syndrome and coeliac disease been demonstrated, with a frequency well above that of the general population. Actually, its prevalence ranges from 0.8 per cent (Simila and Kokkonen 1990) to 4.7 per cent (Castro et al. 1993) in Down syndrome, versus 0.012 per cent to 0.43 per cent in nontrisomic persons (Stenhammar et al. 1993).

Coeliac disease, or gluten intolerance, in its typical, rather uncommon form, is a severe disease developing in early childhood, after the introduction of gluten into the diet. It manifests with diarrhoea, bulky stools, prominent abdomen, and poor thriving. At present, more frequent, atypical or moderate forms are found, appearing late in childhood or in adolescence and showing scarce or absent intestinal manifestations, hypovitaminosis, anaemia, stunted growth. Silent forms are also observed. IgG and IgA gliadin antibodies have been considered a reliable and simple screening test, in order to detect subjects eligible for intestinal biopsy, substituting the more complex and inaccurate xylose test. The first investigations of gliadin antibodies (AGAs) in Down syndrome clearly showed an excess of positive results not confirmed by bioptic data. IgGAGAs, less specific, but more sensitive, are even more often positive (Storm 1990). A more reliable, highly specific screening test is the antiendomysium immunofluorescence test, now almost universally substituting gliadin antibodies. We studied 113 persons with Down syndrome for coeliac disease and found elevated values of IgGAGAs in 48 per cent, of IgAAGAs in 22.1 per cent and of EMA in 6.2 per cent. Four symptomatic patients, AGA- and EMA-positive, were affected by coeliac disease (3.5%): in three AGA- and EMA-positive subjects, permission for intestinal biopsy was refused, while in two AGA-positive, EMA-negative children, the intestinal mucosa was normal (Bonamico et al. 1996). The establishment of a gluten-free diet is the actual therapy and leads to a complete recovery from the disease. The pathogenesis of coeliac disease is still controversial. Recent studies ascribe the responsibility of the mucosal damage to an abnormal immune response to gliadin (Marsh 1992).

Muscular and orthopaedic anomalies are well known in Down syndrome. Muscular hypotonia and joint hyperlaxity are almost constant. Flat foot, genu valgum, and patella instability are the main causes of walking problems, even of severe static troubles such as scoliosis. Prevention is necessary and is feasible through an early and correct mobilisation, an active life, associated with sport activities. The clinical significance of atlantoaxial instability has received specific attention in recent years. Its prevalence is elevated in Down syndrome (10-15%), but is usually asymptomatic (Pueschel and Scola 1987). An increased risk of subluxation and dislocation exists after cervical traumas or abrupt head movements, with neurological complications occurring by cervical cord compression. Dislocation can produce quadriplegia with incontinence or paraplegia that may have a sudden onset or can be preceded by head tilt, abnormal staggering gait and the emergence of neurological signs. Diagnosis is confirmed by X-rays, that demonstrate a distance superior to 5 mm between the anterior aspect of the odontoid process and the posterior margin of the anterior arch of the atlas. Magnetic Resonance Imaging or Computerized Tomographic scans are also useful tools for diagnostic purposes. Children at risk should not be allowed to practise somersaulting, trampolining or similar activities. For symptomatic cases, vertebral fusion is the preferred surgical method (Aicardi 1992).

Dental anomalies are a common problem and often their solution is not an easy task. Moreover, objective difficulties found in visiting and specifically treating children and adults with intellectual disabilities lead to underestimation of actual buccal disorders. A peculiar oral and dental anatomy, developmental anomalies and malocclusion are frequent, while caries seems to be rarer than in normal children. If oral hygiene is poor, gingivitis and periodontal disease are likely to occur, leading to early and total tooth loss. Dental control should be constant from infancy and for the whole life. Accurate orthodontic help should be available, in order to avoid the depressing consequences of dental decay (Lowe 1990).

Sexual maturation is similar to that of the general population. In males, testicular volume and penis dimensions in puberty reach normal values. Cryptorchidism is common and should be corrected early in life, because of the risk of malignant degeneration in adulthood. In females, the development of secondary sex characters follows a regular pattern. Menses are regular. Fertility is reduced in females: only a small number of pregnancies has been observed, resulting in both normal and trisomic babies. Males are almost invariably sterile (only one case of fatherhood has been reported). Since integration is becoming more and more frequent, adolescents must be prepared for a sexually active life. Contraception can be provided in particular cases.

Impaired mental ability and delayed psychomotor development are constant and show a wide range of ultimate attainment that can to some extent be positively influenced by present educational strategies. Neuropsychiatric problems become prevalent with age, including seizures. In adults, there is a constant, though variable, decline of intelligence. A reduction in thought elaboration ability, in particular abstract thought and logical performance, is likely to occur with advancing age, but earlier than in normal persons. Characteristic of ageing in Down syndrome is also the dementia, showing striking similarities with Alzheimer disease and appearing in a number of subjects after the age of 50 years. Clinically, the affected persons show deterioration of mental and emotional responses, apathy or excitement, irritability, temper tantrums, loss of previously acquired vocabulary and a decline in personal habits of cleanliness. The progression is often very rapid. Seizures can be an early sign of Alzheimer disease. No therapy is known at present. Recent investigations suggest that most adults with Down syndrome undergo normal, albeit probably precocious ageing and that they may be at lower risk for Alzheimer disease than previously supposed (Devenny et al. 1996). It is possible that early intensive rehabilitation and social inclusion are beneficial in slowing mental deterioration and ageing.

In conclusion, a thorough knowledge of the natural history of Down syndrome, of the malformations and of the diseases that can be most frequently associated with it, is of paramount importance both for practical purposes, ie, for correct prevention and treatment, and for more basic studies, evaluating phenotype-genotype correlations. Actually, investigations of the last few years have developed medical and rehabilitative strategies that have had beneficial effects on physical and social aspects of persons with Down syndrome, increasing their life duration and favouring social insertion, in short, offering them a better quality of life.

References

Aicardi J (1992) Diseases of the nervous system in childhood. London: Mac Keith Press.

Anneren G, Gustavson KH, Sara V (1993) Normalised growth velocity in children with Down's syndrome during growth hormone therapy. Journal of Intellectual Disability Research 37: 381-7.

Baird PA, Sadovnick AD (1988) Life expectancy in Down syndrome adults. Lancet 2: 1354-6.

Barreca A, Rasore-Quartino A, Acutis MS (1994) Assessment of growth hormone insulin like growth factor-I axis in Down's syndrome. Journal of Endocrinological Investigation 17: 431-6.

Bonamico M, Rasore-Quartino A, Mariani P (1996) Down syndrome and coeliac disease: Usefulness of antigliadin and antiendomysium antibodies. Acta Paediatrica 85: 1503-5.

Carmi R, Boughman JA, Ferencz C (1992) Endocardial cushion defect: Further studies of 'isolated' versus 'syndromic' occurrence. American Journal of Medical Genetics 43: 569-75.

Castells S, Torrado C, Bastian W (1992) Growth hormone deficiency in Down's syndrome children. Journal of Intellectual Disability Research 36: 29-43.

Castro M, Criná A, Papadatou B (1993) Down's syndrome and celiac disease: The prevalence of high IgA-antigliadin antibodies and HLA-DR and DQ antigens in trisomy 21. Journal of Pediatric Gastroenterologic Nutrition 16: 265-8.

Cominetti M, Rasore-Quartino A, Acutis MS, Vignola G (1985) Neonato con sindrome di Down e leucemia mieloide acuta. Difficoltá diagnostiche tra forma maligna e sindrome mieloproliferativa. Pathologica 77: 625-30.

Creutzig U, Ritter J, Vormoor J (1996) Myelodysplasia and acute myelogenous leukemia in Down's syndrome. A report of 40 children of the AML-BFM Study Group. Leukemia 10: 1677-86.

Devenny DA, Silverman WP, Hill AL (1996). Normal ageing in adults with Down's syndrome: a longitudinal study. Journal of Intellectual Disability Research 40: 208-21.

Epstein CJ (1995) Down syndrome. In Scriver A, Beaudet AL, Sly WS, Valle D (eds), The Metabolic and Molecular Basis of Inherited Disease. New York: McGraw Hill.

Fabris N, Mocchegiani E, Amadio L (1984) Thymic hormone deficiency in normal ageing and Down's syndrome: Is there a primary failure of the thymus? Lancet 1: 983-6.

Forni GL, Rasore-Quartino A, Acutis MS, Strigini P (1990) Incidence of bronchial asthma in Down syndrome. Journal of Pediatrics 116: 487.

Fort P, Lifschitz F, Bellisario R (1984) Abnormalities of thyroid function in infants with Down syndrome. Journal of Pediatrics 58: 893-7.

Garrè ML, Relling MV, Kalwinsky D (1987) Pharmacokinetics and toxicity of methotrexate in children with Down's syndrome and acute lymphocytic leukemia. Journal of Pediatrics 111: 606-12.

Goldhaber SZ, Brown WD, St John Sutton MG (1987) High frequency of mitral valve prolapse and aortic regurgitation among asymptomatic adults with Down's syndrome. JAMA 258: 1793-5.

Korenberg JR, Kawashima H, Pulst SM (1990) Molecular definition of a region of chromosome 21 that causes features of the Down syndrome phenotype. American Journal of Human Genetics 47: 236.

Korenberg JR, Chen XN, Schipper R (1994) Down syndrome phenotypes: the consequences of chromosomal imbalance. Proceedings of the National Academy of Science, USA 91: 4997-5001.

Lowe O (1990) Dental problems In Van Dyke DC, Lang DJ, Heide F (eds) Clinical Perspectives in the Management of Down Syndrome. New York: Springer Verlag. pp. 72-9.

Marsh MN (1992) Gluten, major histocompatibility complex and the small intestine. A molecular and immunobiological approach to the spectrum of gluten sensitivity (celiac sprue). Gastroenterology 102: 330-54.

Miller M, Cosgriff JM (1983) Hematologic abnormalities in newborns with Down's syndrome. Journal of Medical Genetics 16: 173-8.

Pueschel SM, Scola FH (1987) Atlantoaxial instability in individuals with Down syndrome: epidemiologic, radiographic and clinical studies. Pediatrics 80: 555-60.

Rasore-Quartino A, Cominetti M (1994) Clinical follow-up of adolescents and adults with Down syndrome. In Nadel L, Rosenthal D (eds) Down Syndrome: Living and Learning in the Community. New York: Wiley-Liss. pp. 238-45.

Rosner F, Lee SL (1972) Down's syndrome and acute leukemia: Myeloblastic or lymphoblastic. Report of forty-three cases and review of the literature. American Journal of Medicine 53: 203-14.

Simila S, Kokkonen J (1990) Coexistence of coeliac disease and Down syndrome. American Journal on Mental Retardation 95: 120-22.

Spicer RL (1984) Cardiovascular disease in Down syndrome. Pediatric Clinics of North America 31: 1331-43.

Stenhammar, L, Asher H, Cavell B (1993) Is the incidence of childhood coeliac disease in Sweden still raising? Acta Paediatrica 82: 1056.

Storm W (1990) Prevalence and diagnostic significance of gliadin antibodies in children with Down syndrome. European Journal of Pediatric 149: 833-4.

Ugazio AG, Maccario R, Notarangelo LD, Burgio GR (1990) Immunology of Down syndrome: a review. American Journal of Medical Genetics, Supplement 7: 204-12.

Weinstein HS (1978) Congenital leukemia and the neonatal myeloproliferative disorders associated with Down's syndrome. Clinical Haematology 7: 147-56.

Chapter 15
Prenatal Diagnosis of Down Syndrome: From Surprise to Certainty

ALBERTO FORTUNY

Introduction

During the last few decades, developments in access to the foetus 'in utero' by noninvasive as well as invasive technologies for the prenatal detection of foetal anomalies and genetic diseases, has made possible the diagnosis of Down syndrome (DS) long before the baby is born.

Although the precise number of human chromosomes had been established (Tjio and Levan 1956) and the nature of the chromosome disorder involved in Down syndrome was known for many years (Lejeune et al. 1959), cytogenetic technology for successful culture and analysis of foetal cells had not been developed, despite the fact that acquisition of amniotic fluid (amniocentesis) to monitor pregnancies with Rh isoimmunization had been introduced by Bevis in 1952.

The first attempts to use amniotic fluid cells for genetic diagnosis were made to disclose foetal sex in pregnancies at risk for X-linked diseases, by determining sex chromatin (Barr body) in foetal cells. However, it was not until the mid 1960s that successful culture of amniotic cells to perform cytogenetic analysis was made possible (Steele and Breg 1956) and shortly after, in 1967, the first prenatal diagnosis of Down syndrome was reported by Jacobson and Barter. Rapid diffusion of amniocentesis during the second trimester of pregnancy for the diagnosis of genetic disease took place in the USA and Europe, after the first series of cases providing evidence of its relative safety and accuracy for prenatal genetic diagnosis were reported.

Additional milestones in the development of prenatal diagnosis have been the support provided by the introduction of ultrasound imaging technology in modern obstetrics, particularly the introduction of high resolution real time ultrasound with improving image definition, making access to representative cells of the foetus from the intrauterine environment safer for the foetus and the mother.

In the 1980s new laboratory and technical progress made it possible to anticipate foetal genetic diagnosis starting from weeks 16-17, as was done by amniocentesis, to the first trimester. This came about by obtaining cells from the placenta thus avoiding the entrance to the amniotic cavity. The proper processing of trophoblastic cells, actively dividing at these early stages of pregnancy and present in small fragments of this tissue, make it possible to provide extraembryonic material adequate for cytogenetic and molecular diagnosis. Ultrasound-guided procedures for chorionic villus sampling (CVS) were thus made possible and its relative safety, when properly performed in experienced centres, has by now been tested in large series, proving to be advantageous for earlier diagnosis.

Prenatal Counselling in Prenatal Diagnosis

Prenatal diagnosis must be understood as a process involving a number of activities, and not just an isolated medical act. It begins and ends with a process of communication between the mother or couple and professionals involved in a multidisciplinary approach, and is intended to provide early, precise and understandable information of potential genetic risks for the foetus, offering diagnostic options and facilitating informed attitudes and decisions.

Preconceptional and prenatal reproductive and genetic counselling are essential parts of current prenatal diagnosis strategies (Table 15.1), and may be followed by application of other resources for screening and diagnostic purposes.

Table 15.1 Requirements for prenatal diagnosis strategies

Counselling:
   Preconceptional for primary prevention
   Postconceptional (prenatal)
Detection of risk factors
Assessment and information
Offer of options :
   Screening resources
   Diagnostic procedures

Some Epidemiological Facts

The prevalence of Down syndrome in live newborns has been estimated overall at 1.5 per 1,000. There is a well-established universal relationship between maternal ageing and increasing risk of meiotic nondisjunction which accounts for over 95 per cent of the newborns affected with Down syndrome. This is the reason why maternal age has been the epidemiological risk criterion most commonly used for offering a prenatal diagnostic test, and the prevalence of Down syndrome in a given pregnant population will depend on its maternal age distribution. At the present time, data for estimation of epidemiological risk based on figures for maternal age and prevalence at birth, or in the second trimester of pregnancy are available from large series of amniocentesis. A higher prevalence in the second trimester than at birth is well substantiated and explained by the significant spontaneous foetal loss of Down syndrome and other aneuploidies during the first and second half of pregnancy.

Although an influence of paternal age on the occurrence of Down syndrome has not been proven, due to the lack of large enough age-discordant series, there is some evidence provided by donor insemination registries showing an increase from 1.4/1,000 at paternal age under 35 years, rising to 2.3 at 35-39 and to 4.1/1,000 for age over 40 (Jalbert 1996).

The offering of amniocentesis to pregnant women at 35 years and over has been mainly based on a balance estimate of the risk of foetal loss involved by performing the procedure and the risk of a particular pregnancy to result in Down syndrome based on the epidemiological maternal age-linked risk. Other less common indications have been the existence of a previous child with Down syndrome and the presence of parental balanced translocations involving chromosome 21.

Over the last decade a growing trend of increasing maternal age of mothers giving birth has been observed in most industrialised countries in Europe and in the USA, more so in urban than in rural populations. With the introduction and availability of prenatal diagnosis, a growing demand for this testing has been observed and it is likely that an undetermined proportion of women, knowing that a reassuring diagnosis is now possible, may deliberately postpone pregnancies for some time.

Data from our unit, active in reproductive and prenatal counselling for over 20 years, and including nearly 22,000 consultations up to 1995 (Table 15.2), show an increasing trend in demand, and the proportion of those related to maternal age or other risk for Down syndrome (Table 15.3). It must be noted that in a significant proportion of those consulting for advanced maternal age, other risk factors were detected which would have gone undetected without proper previous assessment and which would have significantly changed or modified the diagnostic process (Table 15.4).

Screening Strategies for Down Syndrome

Some of the problems presently facing the prenatal diagnosis of Down syndrome relate to the fact that invasive procedures, either second trimester amniocentesis or CVS, although considered acceptably safe and highly accurate, are not exempt from risk, although low, of pregnancy loss. On the other hand, if applied only to women older than 35 years old, which may represent some 10 per cent of the pregnant population, a large proportion of pregnancies, for example the remaining 90 per cent, with significantly lowered risk as maternal age decreases but still with some risk, will be denied the benefit of the diagnosis and timely information.

Table 15.2 Evolving rate of prenatal counselling 1975-95*

Five year-intervals and single year 1995	
Total 1975-95	21352
1975-79	368
1980-84	2051
1985-89	6883
1990-94	9225
1995	2825

*Prenatal diagnosis and reproductive counselling unit, Hospital Clinic, University of Barcelona.

Table 15.3 Request for counselling related to Down syndrome risk

Advanced maternal age	10.011 (46.8%)
Familial Down syndrome	803 (3.8%)
Anxiety 'sine cause' related to D.S	727 (3.4%)
Total	(11.541 of 21.372) (54%)

Table 15.4 Consultation of pregnancies for advanced maternal age, and other risk factors detected

Total	852 (8.5%)
Genetic	295 (3%)
Teratogen	49 (0.5%)
Multifactorial	20 (0.2%)
Unidentified mental retardation	60 (0.6%)
Other*	428 (4.3%)

*Monogenic, consanguinity, repeated spontaneous abortion, sterility of unknown cause.

Although this debate has strong financial and cost-benefit implications, the issue of more accurately selecting those pregnancies in which to offer diagnostic procedures in order to minimize unnecessary invasive procedures has been faced, by means of better selecting those pregnancies at 'higher risk' of being affected by trisomy 21 amongst all pregnant women.

Up to the mid 1980s, the only screening criteria used were asking the mother for her age and establishing the maternal age-based risk. A change came about after the finding in 1984 that maternal serum levels of a foetal protein (Alphafoetoprotein or AFP), whose increased levels had been used for some years for the detection of open neural tube defects, were on average significantly lower in pregnancies affected by Down syndrome than in unaffected pregnancies. The use of this marker in screening during the second trimester proved valuable for detection purposes, and was the first step in the development of the present strategies.

Shortly thereafter, other markers, such as the rise of maternal serum levels of chorionic gonadotrophin (HCG), a protein produced by the placenta, and lowering of unconjugated estriol, an esteroid produced in large amounts during pregnancy, were later tested and added in order to increase detection rates, with the use of a pre-established cut-off of risk value (commonly above 1:250 to 1:270). At the present time these markers, particularly AFP and HCG in maternal serum, have been extensively tested in retrospective and prospective large series and have proven to be capable, in combination with maternal age, of more than doubling detection rates in screening unselected populations of pregnant women (as compared to the isolated use of maternal age over 35 as a screening criterion) by offering an invasive procedure based on a more precise risk, for the prenatal cytogenetic diagnosis.

This test, inexpensive and simple to perform, has by now been widely introduced and offered in the second trimester (between weeks 14–17). It must be done by experienced laboratories, with monitoring of the results, and adjustment for factors which may modify the serum values of the markers. It must also be based on pre-established norms for each week of unaffected pregnancies, since normal serum values of the markers change with the progress of gestation, and deviations from the norm are calculated as multiples of the median values for each gestational week in unaffected pregnancies.

Significant progress is being made in the application of other serum markers during the first trimester of pregnancy, from weeks 9 to 12, with promising results. In this regard a specific placental protein (Pregnancy associated placental protein A or PAPP-A) and a subunit of hCG (free-ß hCG) appear to be the choice for first trimester screening of Down syndrome and, therefore, to offer earlier diagnostic procedures such as chorionic villus sampling (CVS).

Also, with the improvement of ultrasound definition, some foetal structural changes in the first and early second trimester have been found to be more commonly observed in Down syndrome than in unaffected pregnacies. An increase in thickness of the foetal neck (nuchal translucency or nuchal fold), which can be precisely measured from the tenth week, is at present considered an ultrasound marker which is being used as a noninvasive test, in unselected pregnancies at any maternal age, to better offer an invasive test for diagnosis. It is likely that, with the use of both biochemical maternal serum analyses and ultrasound, selection of pregnancies to offer invasive diagnostic testing will be significantly improved.

Other ultrasound findings commonly associated with Down syndrome, such as congenital heart defects, particularly atrial-ventricular septal defects and less commonly duodenal atresia, can be detected in the second trimester of pregnancy.

Invasive Procedures for Prenatal Cytogenetic Diagnosis

At the present time amniocentesis and chorionic villus sampling are the common procedures offered for foetal cytogenetic diagnosis.

Amniocentesis, still the most widely used method from the fifteenth week of pregnancy, involves an outpatient transabdominal procedure without the need of sedation or analgesia. Accumulated experience in prospective control and randomized trials has estimated an increase in foetal loss due to the procedure of 0.5–0.8 per cent over the background spontaneous loss, in the context of a highly accurate sampling for cytogenetic diagnosis. Relative disadvantages are the long period for culture and cytogenetic evaluation which may extend from two to three weeks, so the diagnosis is commonly not available earlier than at 17 to 18 weeks.

New developments in molecular cytogenetics are presently available, such as the methods of fluorescence in situ hybridization (FISH) using specific probes for the chromosomes most commonly involved including chromosome 21. These can be used in nondividing cells (interphase cells) present in either amniotic fluid or CVS, and provide evidence for the presence of fluorescent signals identifiable as the presence of the extra chromosome. This provides a preliminary report in a very short time in nondividing cells and, although it is not used as a definitive diagnosis, it can provide an early assurance of normality, to be confirmed in metaphase analysis of cultured cells.

Chorionic villi sampling is performed as a first trimester procedure from the tenth week and it may be extended up to the fifteenth week. It can be done by either a transcervical or transabdominal procedure. Although its accuracy is high, in some 1 per cent of cases a confined abnormality in trophoblastic cells is observed that is not present in the foetus. However, when the diagnosis in CVS is of nonmosaic trisomy 21 the predictive value is virtually 100 per cent. When other rare trisomies are found, amniocentesis must be carried out for confirmation, but this may be needed in only 1 per cent of the CVS performed.

CVS has obvious advantages for an earlier diagnosis and short reporting time which may be available within a few days of sampling.

Conclusion

It can be said that prenatal diagnosis is now possible through procedures that are both safe and accurate when the pregnancies are properly selected. The change in recent years has been from the surprise of knowing that the baby has Down syndrome at the time of birth, to the precise knowledge and certainty of this fact during pregnancy long before birth.

The advantages provided by this information to the mother or the couple can be debated. However, there is evidence that this early and precise information, provided in the calm environment of dialogue with the prospective mother, can facilitate the adjustment to a new situation much better than suddenly knowing it after the uneasy process of a delivery. This anticipated certainty can be seen as a favourable situation for future of mother-child bonding. In addition it will permit more adequate perinatal care and, if an additional anomaly such as congenital heart defect or bowel atresia is known to be present, it will allow better neonatal anticipation for proper care and treatment.

References

Bevis D (1952) The antenatal prediction of hemolitic disease of the newborn. Lancet: 395-8.

Jacobson C, Barter R (1967) Intrauterine diagnosis and management of genetic defects. American Journal of Obstetrics and Gynecology 99: 796-807.

Jalbert P (1996) Down syndrome incidence and paternal age. Screening News: 3-5.

Lejeune J, Gautier M, Turpin R (1959). Etude des chromosomes somatiques de neuf enfants mongoliens. Comptes Rendus de l'Académie des Sciences de Paris 248: 1721-2.

Steele M, Breg W (1956). Chromosome analysis of human amniotic-fluid cells. Lancet: 385-7.

Tjio JH, Levan A (1956) The chromosome number in man. Hereditas 42: 1-6.

Chapter 16
Ethical Issues Pertaining to Prenatal Diagnosis of Down Syndrome

SIEGFRIED M PUESCHEL

Introduction

Although prenatal genetic counseling has been available sporadically since the early part of this century, new emerging techniques developed during the past few decades including amniocentesis, chorionic villus sampling, ultrasound examinations, and others have revolutionized prenatal diagnosis of genetic and chromosomal disorders. Since the introduction of these procedures, genetic counsellors have been able to provide more accurate information to many prospective parents regarding the outcome of the pregnancy. Instead of discussing general probabilities of risk, the genetic counselor can often now tell parents whether the foetus does or does not have a specific genetic or chromosomal disorder.

The advances in prenatal diagnosis may have significant legal implications insofar as a physician may be liable for negligent genetic counseling or failure to test for a specific genetic disorder. For example, the parents of an affected child may allege that the physician failed to inform them that they were at an increased risk of having a child with a genetic or chromosomal disorder and that specific tests were available that could have detected the disorder. Some parents have sued physicians who had neglected to perform a specific prenatal examination or incorrectly interpreted the results of prenatally performed tests that deprived the parents of the opportunity to prevent the birth of an affected child. During the past decade numerous court cases have been publicized in the USA in which parents have been successful in suing physicians because of negligent genetic counselling resulting in 'wrongful birth' of an affected child (Fleisher 1987).

Therefore, 'good medical practice' dictates that physicians advise parents of the availability of various prenatal diagnostic procedures if the foetus seems to be at an increased risk. Physicians involved in prenatal counseling should obtain a detailed family history, employ available 'standard' screening procedures, and provide pertinent genetic information so that parents can make well-informed decisions. If physicians do not pursue such lines of action, litigations may be forthcoming if an affected infant is born. Physicians who are not familiar with specific genetic concerns that should be considered during prenatal counselling should make referrals to professionals who are knowledgeable in this field and are willing to counsel parents appropriately.

Generally speaking, a genetic screening procedure should identify by means of a safe, simple, and inexpensive method a disorder that has important health implications and is amenable to treatment. However, at the present time, some of the screening procedures lack high sensitivity and specificity, require a certain expertise, and are often costly (Pueschel 1987). Moreover, there are only a few genetic disorders in which intrauterine treatment will prevent significant medical problems in the genetically affected child. For the majority of chromosomal and genetic disorders identified during prenatal diagnostic screening, no effective therapy is available and often 'therapeutic' abortion is the only recommendation that is provided to the parents.

The Pros and Cons of Abortion

Proponents of prenatal diagnosis and selective abortion if an affected foetus has been identified point out that (a) it benefits the individual woman and her family, (b) it also benefits society because such procedures have an eugenic effect in eliminating defective genes from the gene pool, (c) it reduces the financial burden to society, (d) it is preventive medicine, (e) it increases the quality of life for the family, and (f) the foetus has a right to be born healthy.

The question arises, what are the underlying factors implying that termination of pregnancy, when an affected foetus has been identified, is the appropriate course of action? We also have to ask, is it possible that our forefathers' attitudes and past approaches to the care of people with handicapping conditions are still influencing present-day thinking? It is well known that in the past, persons with Down syndrome were felt to be severely mentally retarded and that there was little or no potential for their productive employment resulting in substantial costs to taxpayers (Scheerenberger 1983). Moreover, in past decades it was common practice to institutionalize individuals with Down syndrome and other developmental disabilities. At that time, the pertinent teaching in medical schools and residency training programmes adhered to such philosophy, indicating that persons with Down syndrome did not fit in society and that they were better off among their 'own kind' in residential facilities.

Therefore, it is not surprising that when prevention of mental retardation was emphasized during the past few decades and when amniocentesis and other procedures became available, many professionals felt that 'therapeutic' abortion of identified affected foetuses could prevent genetic disorders such as Down syndrome. Stein et al. (1973) suggested that 'almost total prevention of Down syndrome could be achieved by screening all pregnant women using amniocentesis and selective abortion'. These authors indicated that 'the ideology of public health endorses total prevention as a desirable objective; for a condition with a rising prevalence like Down syndrome this objective is better achieved sooner than later'. In the attempt to convince the scientific community of 'the enormous benefits of such prevention efforts', the authors maintained that 'a screening programme must offer termination to all those in whom the chromosomal anomaly is detected'. Stein et al. also mentioned that 'the cost of screening mothers over 30 years of age is certainly less than that of caring for cases of Down syndrome' and that 'the lifelong care of severely retarded persons is so burdensome in almost every human dimension that no preventive programme is likely to outweigh the burden'. Stein and Polkes (1973) also stated 'it is clear that many parents especially those in high risk categories, for instance mothers over 40 years and older, would choose to abort a mongoloid child rather than let it come to term'.

Other professionals approached the prevention of the birth of a child with Down syndrome from a purely economic viewpoint using cost-benefit analysis. Conley (1985) claimed that there is a 'loss of output' either because persons with Down syndrome are unemployable or they die prematurely. Moreover, Conley indicated that an excess of educational and residential care expenses would make prenatal identification of a child with Down syndrome and subsequent abortion economically 'attractive'. He estimated the social cost of Down syndrome to be about $3,621,000,000, whereas the prevention of Down syndrome including amniocentesis, chromosomal analysis, counseling, and abortion amounted only to $33,000,000. According to this author, such cost-benefit analysis shows that society would save money if foetuses with Down syndrome were selectively aborted.

Fletcher (1973) advocates screening, 'compulsory if necessary', to locate as many affected foetuses as possible. He defends screening as 'no more an invasion of privacy than contact tracing in the treatment of a venereal disease'. His position is that foetuses with severe defects have a 'lesser moral claim on the mother than normal children' because they are less likely to 'respond to the promise of becoming a person in the community of persons'.

McCormick (1974) asks, where should one draw the line to determine humanity? He argues that the potentiality for human relationship is the requirement that must be met, and asserts that 'life is not a value to be preserved in and for itself, but it is a value to be preserved precisely for other values'.

Because current advances in medical treatment have allowed more genetically diseased persons to survive and reproduce, some professionals are afraid that this trend would allow the number of 'bad genes' in our society to increase causing a 'gene pool crisis' (McCormick 1974). According to this author, one method of reversing this trend and saving or even improving future generations is to selectively abort affected foetuses. Yet, it has been estimated that the actual change in the gene pool's composition due to selective abortion is very small (Motulsky 1974; Murphy and Chase 1975).

Although many of the prenatal diagnostic procedures have significantly contributed to the advances in human genetics and many of them have been hailed as major breakthroughs, it has been questioned whether the identification and subsequent abortion of genetically defective foetuses indeed constitute 'real progress' (LeJeune, personal communications). Of course, prenatal diagnosis has many potential beneficial uses, in particular if therapy for the affected foetus is available and/or if parents can be counseled with regard to future reproductive risks. These justifiable uses, however, should not be overshadowed by allowing them to become strictly an exercise of selective abortion.

Whereas proponents of prenatal diagnosis and termination of pregnancy emphasize that each child should have a right to be born 'healthy', many parents consider amniocentesis and chorionic villus sampling a waste of efforts since they would not opt to abort anyhow. For example, Keiler Paul (1987), who gave birth to a child with Down syndrome, expressed her views as follows: 'On the one hand we wanted and planned this child and didn't think we had the right to be choosy as to say we will keep it only if it's up to spec'. She continued, 'we really never know what we're getting when we elect to create another individual. And why assume that a child with a handicap will be a negative experience? For all the joy and richness they have brought into our lives, I am grateful to have all our children with all their weaknesses and strengths'.

When Pearl S Buck (1973) reflected on the meaning of her retarded child, she said, 'could it have been possible for me to have had foreknowledge of her thwarted life, would I have wanted an abortion? With full knowledge of anguish and despair, the answer is no, I would not. Even in full knowledge I would have chosen life and this is for two reasons: first I fear the power of choice over life or death that is at human hands. I see no human being whom I could ever trust with such power. Human wisdom, human integrity are not great enough. Secondly, my child's life has not been meaningless. She has indeed brought comfort and practical help to many people who are parents of retarded children or are themselves handicapped. True, she has done it through me, yet without her I would not have had the means of learning how to accept the inevitable sorrow and how to make that acceptance useful to others.' Pearl S Buck continues, 'in this world, where cruelty prevails in so many aspects of our lives, I would not add the weight of choice to kill rather to let live. A retarded child, a handicapped person brings his own gift to life, even to the life of normal human beings. That gift is comprehended in the lessons of patience, understanding, and mercy, lessons which we all need to relive and to practise with one another, whatever we are. For this gift bestowed upon me by a helpless child, I give my thanks.'

According to Pearl S. Buck's philosophy, the current practice of prenatal diagnosis and selective abortion is threatening basic human rights. The assumption that children with Down syndrome will be significantly retarded or that they will never enjoy the delights of physical or intellectual achievements as 'normal' persons do is not a valid reason to recommend pregnancy termination if the foetus has been found to have Down syndrome.

Although many geneticists consider Down syndrome to be a clear-cut case calling for abortion, many parents feel that to determine that a foetus with Down syndrome should be aborted is to make a social judgement about the place of individuals with developmental disabilities in society. It is possible to judge disability or deviation from the norm medically, but to determine that this deviation constitutes a significant handicap is make a social judgement.

It has been argued that it is 'more just and causes less suffering to the foetus to abort it rather than allowing it to suffer pain and illness' (Neel 1967). This argument must be considered invalid because of its inherent paternalism and because of its incorrect assumptions relative to Down syndrome.

In addition, the argument that it is unjust to society to allow more children with disabilities to be born is especially vulnerable to the charge of intolerance. Moreover, some other professionals indicate that since approximately 70 to 80 per cent of foetuses with Down syndrome are spontaneously miscarried, why not help 'Mother Nature' and get rid of the remaining foetuses with this chromosomal disorder. Such thinking does not take into consideration the significant difference of a miscarriage and the active removal of the foetus from the uterus.

Many geneticists stress the fact that most of the prenatal diagnoses will reveal a normal foetus and hence serve to reassure anxious couples. This reassurance rationale can be tested by asking whether any woman could have amniocentesis if she had no intention of having an abortion in the event of an abnormality or just to make sure that the foetus she carries is 'normal'. Considering the limited resources in many parts of the world, the answer to both questions frequently will be in the negative.

Similarly, the argument that prenatal diagnosis saves lives by preventing abortions also depends on the acceptance of selective abortion. The interest here is not in saving lives of all foetuses by preventing all abortions, but only in saving the lives of 'normal' foetuses by preventing them from being aborted. Thus, the entire line of reasoning depends on the acceptance of abortion of foetuses with significant abnormalities.

For some people the justification for selective abortion rests upon the hypothetical judgement as to the life of and the value of that life to the potential infant. Many parents see human life as precious and reject the assumption of a life's lack of worth and value as a justification for its termination. Other parents feel that an IQ score is a demeaning measure of human potential and that the assumption of the presence of mental retardation in the child with Down syndrome is not a justification for aborting that foetus.

Concerning cost-benefit analyses which often indicate that society would save money if foetuses with Down syndrome were to be selectively aborted, it is of note that these studies usually focus on the cost of the tests versus the cost of the care of individuals with developmental disabilities. The cost of the screening tests (alphafoetoprotein and triple test), confirmatory tests (chorionic villus sampling, amniocentesis and chromosomal analysis), genetic counseling, and termination of pregnancy is usually underestimated and the cost of the education and long-term care (institutionalization) is often exaggerated (Conley 1985). Today, the majority of individuals with Down syndrome will never be institutionalized and many of them will be gainfully employed and will become productive citizens.

When a condition is considered to be eligible for prenatal diagnosis, it may imply that persons who are affected are undesirable or unfit. Simply offering prenatal diagnosis for certain conditions such as for the identification of foetuses with chromosomal abnormalities and not for others may suggest that it is ethically acceptable to perform such tests and to terminate a pregnancy if an abnormality is found. Actually, there is no evidence that society would significantly improve if the incidence of children born with this chromosomal disorder were to be reduced through prenatal diagnosis and abortion (Fost 1981).

Concern has also been expressed by parents that prenatal diagnosis of a chromosomal disorder such as Down syndrome may affect attitudes toward living persons with this condition. Moreover, public support for programmes to wipe out or significantly diminish the occurrence of a particular condition may undermine the support for treatment of persons already born with this condition. Also, public awareness of reducing the incidence of 'abnormal births' may unintentionally bring pressure to bear on the women who carry such a pregnancy to term (Fost 1981).

Genetic Counseling

Many questions arise about providing appropriate genetic counseling to parents who have been told that their foetus has Down syndrome. What kind of information should professionals give the parents, and in what way should this information be communicated? Is it possible for counselors who do not have any direct experience with youngsters with Down syndrome and know about Down syndrome primarily from lectures and from books to give an unbiased portrait of the life of children with Down syndrome? How do counselors discuss with parents the various aspects of medical, intellectual, social, and other issues that are part of the Down syndrome phenotype? And in what ways do counselors' personal attitudes, outlook on life, value systems, and ethical considerations influence the parents' decision-making process?

Counselors must realize that no message provided to parents is value-free. They should never advocate a particular action but should transmit factual information and present alternative points of view.

Parents who are confronted with a profoundly distressing situation such as the diagnosis of Down syndrome in their foetus frequently display impaired decision-making capacity because of prevailing cognitive dysfunction. During this traumatic period, parents are extremely vulnerable to external influences and suggestions. They may not fully understand the presented medical complexities and the long-term implications. Yet, immediate decisions often need to be made in regard to whether the pregnancy should be terminated or continued. Parents are more able to come to a decision if they are afforded access to a range of resources beyond the expertise of a single counselor. For example, other parents who have a child with Down syndrome may provide the distressed parents with a different viewpoint of the life of a child with this chromosomal disorder.

It is paramount that in addition to providing facts and options, genetic counselors focus on positive aspects of caring for a child with Down syndrome. Moreover, they should help parents to cope because the information provided to them can be quite emotionally burdensome. Being told that their foetus has Down syndrome may elicit feelings of guilt, denial, anger, and unforeseen anxieties in parents may become apparent. Sensitive counselors should be attuned to these reactions and should understand the symbolism of behaviour during stressful situations.

Whereas in the past physicians often told parents what actions should be taken, today most counselors use a nondirective approach in their counseling efforts. If factual information, various options, and guidance are sensitively provided by counselors, parents will be able to make independent decisions based upon the knowledge they have gained through the genetic counseling process.

References

Buck PS (1973) The Child who Never Grew. New York: The John Day Company.
Conley RW (1985) Down syndrome: Economic burdens and benefits of prevention. In Dellarco VL, Voytek PE, Hollaender A (eds) Aneuploidy: Etiology and Mechanisms. New York: Plenum. pp. 35-73.
Fleisher LD (1987) Wrongful births. When is there liability for prenatal injury? American Journal of Diseases of Children 141: 1260-5.
Fletcher J (1973) Ethics and euthanasia. American Journal of Nursing 73: 670-5.

Fost N. (1981) Amniocentesis: ethical and psychological issues in prenatal diagnosis. Pediatric Basics 29: 11-15.

Keiler Paul C (1987) Real life thoughts on amniocentesis. Down Syndrome News 11: 51.

McCormick TR (1974) Ethical issues in amniocentesis and abortion. Texas Reports on Biology and Medicine 32: 299-309.

Motulsky A (1974) Brave new world? Science 185: 653-63.

Murphy EA, Chase GA (1975) Principles of Genetic Counseling. Chicago: Year Book Medical Publishers.

Neel JF (1967) Prenatal diagnosis and therapeutic abortion. Perspectives in Biology and Medicine 11: 129-35.

Pueschel SM (1987) Maternal alpha-fetoprotein screening for Down syndrome. New England Journal of Medicine 317: 376-8.

Scheerenberger RC (1983) A History of Mental Retardation. Baltimore, MD: Brookes.

Stein Z, Polkes AV (1973) The prevention of Down's syndrome. Annals of Clinical Research 5: 63-7.

Stein Z, Susser M, Guterman AV (1973) Screening programme for prevention of Down's syndrome. Lancet i: 305-10.

Chapter 17
Down Syndrome and Alzheimer Disease: Variability in Individual Vulnerability

WAYNE SILVERMAN AND HENRYK M WISNIEWSKI

Introduction

Alzheimer disease (AD) is the most common cause of old-age associated dementia (eg, Terry and Katzman 1983). It was first described over 90 years ago (Alzheimer 1907), and the association between Down syndrome (DS) and Alzheimer disease was noted only 22 years later (Struwe 1929). Since that time, numerous studies have confirmed that risk for Alzheimer disease is increased dramatically among adults with Down syndrome, and we have recently reviewed this topic elsewhere (eg, Silverman et al. 1998; Wisniewski and Silverman 1996; Zigman et al. 1994). Despite the fact that both Alzheimer disease and its link with Down syndrome were reported so long ago, we are only now beginning to gain a fundamental understanding of the nature of the extremely complex, age-associated phenomena responsible for this association.

Over the past 15 years, interest in the connection between Down syndrome and Alzheimer disease has intensified for two quite distinct reasons. Because Down syndrome is caused by an alteration in the chromosomes of affected individuals (typically a complete triplication of chromosome 21), groups and individuals concerned about Alzheimer disease hope to gain insights into the genetic mechanisms controlling this progressive and devastating neurodegenerative disease from studies of adults with Down syndrome. Independently, groups and individuals concerned about mental retardation and Down syndrome have recognized that life expectancy for this population has increased dramatically in recent decades (eg, Strauss and Eyman 1996). Therefore, there is an urgent and growing need to develop an understanding of the health risks that are associated with ageing in these individuals. Alzheimer disease is likely to be among the most significant concerns, especially for adults with Down syndrome, and plans must be developed to ensure that needed services will be available and that opportunities for prevention of dementia can be utilized effectively.

We are now reaping the benefits of this interest, and our fundamental understanding of Alzheimer disease and its effect on adults with Down syndrome has been advancing rapidly. Nevertheless, for adults with mental retardation, regardless of its cause, available knowledge is severely limited regarding: (a) factors that determine individual differences in risk for Alzheimer disease; (b) methods for defining objectively the presence of dementia, especially for establishing a diagnosis during early to middle stages of progression; (c) estimates of age-specific incidence (reflecting new cases within the population) and prevalence (reflecting total cases within the population); and (d) descriptions of the profile(s) of clinical progression. This chapter will review the current state of our knowledge regarding these issues, discuss some of the recent developments related more generally to Alzheimer disease, and outline priorities that now need to be addressed to advance our ability to deal effectively with Alzheimer disease and other primary progressive dementias as they affect 'elderly' adults with Down syndrome.

Alzheimer Disease: A Brief Overview

Alzheimer disease is the most common cause of primary progressive dementia affecting elderly people. Alone, it accounts for up to 50 per cent of all cases of late onset dementia, and it appears to contribute to approximately another 30 per cent of cases in combination with other types of brain pathology (Terry and Katzman 1983). Currently, there are no true case registries in place, but it seems clear that prevalence is increasing. This is due to the fact that risk is strongly age-dependent, ever greater numbers of people are living to older and older ages, and extended survival opportunities for affected individuals are being provided by improvements in care. Evans (1990) has suggested that shortly after the turn of the century, as many as 10,000,000 Americans may be affected, and as many as 4,000,000 Americans may be affected currently.

Dementia of the Alzheimer type

Alzheimer disease causes a primary progressive dementia, having direct effects on brain function that result in a worsening clinical picture over time. Treatment for the progressive brain damage caused by Alzheimer disease is not yet available. However, symptomatic treatments can be used to improve quality of life, at least temporarily, and some recently developed medications appear to be effective in slowing the rate of dementia in some cases (see Small et al. 1997).

According to ICD-10 (WHO 1992), dementia in Alzheimer disease is characterized by disturbances in multiple mental functions, among which are memory, thought, orientation, comprehension, calculation, learning capacity, language and/or judgement. The disturbances that are present are not dependent upon clouding of consciousness, and can be accompanied or preceded by changes in emotional control, social behaviour or motivation. Symptoms worsen over time, beginning insidiously with slow progression. Memory impairment is a principal defining feature, and the devastating course of this disease has been well described (eg, Reisberg et al. 1989). The relatively subtle changes in memory typical of the earliest deficits will progress to the point of total dependency, where all self-care, language and motor abilities are lost unless deterioration is interrupted by death due to other causes.

Small et al. (1997) have provided the most recent consensus statement regarding the diagnosis and treatment of Alzheimer disease and related disorders. Several points included in this report are of direct relevance to a discussion of dementia in adults with Down syndrome. First, although dementia among the nonretarded population can be diagnosed on the basis of a general medical exam, diagnostic errors among physicians are still quite common (eg, Callahan et al. 1995; Ryan 1994). This indicates that the diagnosis of dementia is far from straightforward in standard primary practice, even where clear classification criteria have been developed and valid testing methods are broadly available.

Individual differences in abilities preceding the onset of dementia further complicate interpretation of diagnostic assessment results. Small et al. emphasized that evidence of changes in status compared with an individual's previous performance is essential for diagnosis of dementia, and test results at any single point in time are less informative. As an example, Small et al. discussed scores on the Mini-Mental State Examination (Folstein et al. 1975), a well-recognized screen for dementia of the Alzheimer type. Scores indicating 'normal' performance can be obtained for highly educated adults even when cognitive declines are present. Alternatively, scores indicating 'impaired' performance can be obtained for adults with minimal education even though they are experiencing no cognitive loss. Of course, the latter situation has direct relevance to populations with mental retardation and Down syndrome. Therefore, accurate diagnosis of any person presenting with atypical patterns of performance before the suspected onset of dementia depends upon expert assessment. By extension, this would be true for all adults with Down syndrome.

Second, the diagnosis of dementia will usually be based on documentation of patterns of cognitive and functional decline provided by a combination of interviews with knowledgeable informants and direct evaluation. Sophisticated laboratory tests or neuroimaging studies, while recommended by many clinicians and experts, are most frequently used to identify treatable conditions that may be causing the dementia symptoms or comorbid conditions that, when treated, could provide some more or less temporary improvement in overall condition. Thus, for adults with mental retardation and Down syndrome, the quality of diagnosis will depend upon the availability of methods to document significant declines in clinical status. Unfortunately, no consensus yet exists, even among experts, regarding the appropriate clinical procedures, although general agreement has been achieved regarding priority areas for examination and the general strategies to be pursued to document declines over time (eg, Aylward et al. 1997).

Small et al. made a third point that is of particular relevance to the issue of Alzheimer disease as it affects adults with Down syndrome. Clinical practice has now advanced to the point where the diagnosis of Alzheimer disease should be one of inclusion rather than exclusion. Traditionally, Alzheimer disease has only been diagnosed after all other possible causes of dementia symptoms have been ruled out through extensive evaluations (exclusionary diagnosis). However, because the characteristics that differentiate dementia of the Alzheimer type from other conditions, including other primary progressive dementias, have been described with sufficient precision, proper evaluation procedures can provide accuracy levels of approximately 90 per cent with respect to differential diagnosis (eg, Larson et al. 1996). It will not be possible to achieve a comparable level of accuracy in differential diagnosis for adults with mental retardation for some years to come, but this represents a goal to which we can aspire.

Neuropathology

The underlying causes of Alzheimer disease are still unknown. However, a clear pattern of brain changes has been associated with this disease, and multiple forms of neuropathology will occur as the disease process progresses. These include gross atrophy (reduction of brain mass), loss of neurons, loss of synapses, granulovacuolar degeneration, formation of Hirano bodies, amyloid angiopathy, neurofibrillary pathology (including neurofibrillary tangles), and formation of amyloid-ß plaques (Mirra et al. 1994).

Among the multiple types of brain changes seen in Alzheimer disease, accumulations of two microscopic lesions, amyloid-ß plaques and neurofibrillary tangles, are currently employed as diagnostic hallmarks. Amyloid- ß plaques form outside of neurons and occur in several subtypes. Of these, it now appears to be particularly important to differentiate between neuritic plaques, which contain substantial numbers of fibrils, and diffuse plaques, which do not. Disruption of neuron functioning has been associated only with the presence of neuritic plaques, but not with diffuse amyloid-ß deposition (eg, Braak and Braak 1991; Wisniewski et al. 1996). In fact, the impact and significance of diffuse plaque formation is currently uncertain (eg, The National Institute on Aging and Reagan Institute Working Group on Diagnostic Criteria for the Neuropathological Assessment of Alzheimer Disease 1997; Wisniewski and Silverman 1997), and it has been suggested that these lesions may be benign reflections of 'normal' ageing processes (eg, Braak and Braak 1991; Wisniewski et al. 1996), although this is far from certain.

While the multiple types of neuropathological changes associated with Alzheimer disease have been well described, the relationships among these types of brain changes are not yet fully understood. In fact, there persists active debate regarding the fundamental nature of progression. Some scientists have argued that localized neurofibrillary pathology typically begins well before amyloid-ß deposition occurs (eg, Braak and Braak 1997), while others have taken the position that formation of amyloid-ß plaques initiates the cascade of brain changes observed as the disease progresses (eg, Hardy and Higgins 1992). This is only one issue that highlights the fact that current knowledge is imperfect regarding the underlying cause(s) and progression of Alzheimer neuropathology. In fact, a recent supplement to the journal *Neurobiology of Aging* (1997) was devoted exclusively to discussions of current understandings, priorities that need to be addressed through additional research, and development of consensus working diagnostic criteria.

Genetics and other risk factors

Associations between Alzheimer disease and familial susceptibility in relatively rare early onset cases have been recognized for many years, but full appreciation of the relevance of genetic factors is quite recent. Over the past two decades, there has been a revolution taking place in molecular biology and genetics, as illustrated by the Human Genome Project currently mapping the location of literally every gene on every chromosome. These efforts are providing valuable insights into the genetic mechanisms influencing susceptibility to Alzheimer disease.

To date, four genetic loci have been explicitly associated with risk for Alzheimer disease. Two genes, one on chromosome 14 and another on chromosome 1 (presenilin 1 gene and presenilin 2 gene, respectively), have been linked to uncommon forms of Alzheimer disease where expression is particularly aggressive (Levy-Lehad et al. 1995; Rogaev et al. 1995; Sherrington et al. 1995). A third gene, producing amyloid precursor protein (APP), is centrally involved in the mechanism(s) underlying formation of amyloid-ß plaques (eg, Goate et al. 1991), and has been localized on chromosome 21 (eg, Robakis et al. 1987). This gene clearly contributes to the increased risk for Alzheimer disease seen in adults with Down syndrome. Finally, the gene coding for apolipoprotein E (Apo E) has been localized on chromosome 19 (eg, Strittmater et al. 1993), and variation in the three alleles of this gene (Apo ∈-2, -3, -4) is known to affect risk. The presence of Apo ∈-4 is associated with increased vulnerability (Corder et al. 1993; Strittmatter et al. 1993), and Apo ∈-2 is associated with a protective effect (Corder et al. 1994).

Pericak-Vance et al. (1997) recently screened the entire genome for other genetic markers of risk for Alzheimer disease. They found preliminary evidence of involvement for as yet unidentified genes on chromosomes 4, 6, 12 and 20. Thus, while all of the genetic factors involved have clearly not yet been identified, it is already clear that multiple factors have important relevance. These can exert their effects either acting independently or in conjunction with other genetic or environmental factors. Because the onset of Alzheimer disease is, in the vast majority of cases, so late in life, it is clear that gene expression is influenced by factors associated with lifespan development, and therefore it is important to think about individual differences in vulnerability less by whether Alzheimer disease occurs in the absolute sense but rather by its age of onset.

Nongenetic factors also have been related to risk for Alzheimer disease (for discussions see Small et al. 1997; Zigman et al. 1997). Risk seems to be increased with a history of head trauma and lower levels of education, and both of these factors are directly relevant to adults with Down syndrome. Women are at greater risk than men, and this could involve both genetic and environmental factors. Risk among women may be reduced somewhat by oestrogen replacement therapy following menopause, and regular exposure to nonsteroidal anti-inflammatory medications seems to be beneficial regardless of sex, as does treatment with relatively high doses of vitamin E.

Alzheimer Disease and Down Syndrome

The overview of current understandings of Alzheimer disease, though far from complete, provides enough of a framework for discussing the association between this devastating disease and Down syndrome. As mentioned already, there has been a longstanding awareness of this connection (Struwe 1929), but until recently, little serious attention was paid to the relevant observations. Despite the catastrophic effects of Alzheimer disease on affected individuals, there was no compelling public health concern about either Alzheimer disease or its effect on adults with Down syndrome because of the rarity of dementia. Adults, with or without mental retardation, typically did not survive to ages at risk until quite recently, and it is the dramatic increase in life expectancy that has occurred in the second half of the twentieth century that has, with its clear benefits, caused Alzheimer disease and other primary progressive dementias to be the major public health concern that they have become.

For adults with Down syndrome, the size of the subpopulation with Alzheimer disease can be projected employing current estimates of incidence and survival. As an example, in the United States (population of around 260,000,000) there will be approximately 260,000 people with Down syndrome surviving past infancy (eg, Hook 1981). If 55 per cent of these people can now be expected to survive to reach their 55th birthday (eg, Strauss and Eyman 1996), and 45 per cent of these adults develop Alzheimer disease (eg, Zigman et al. 1996), then there could be a US patient population of 75,000 cases. Of course, this is a relatively small number compared to the millions of total cases with Alzheimer disease mentioned earlier (eg, Evans 1990). However, in the context of systems providing services to people with mental retardation, 75,000 adults form a major group of consumers. In fact, only the most populous individual states within the USA serve more than 75,000 total adult consumers of mental retardation/developmental disabilities services (Braddock et al. 1997).

Alzheimer neuropathology among adults with Down syndrome

With extremely few exceptions (eg, Prasher et al. 1998; Visser et al. 1997), adults with Down syndrome dying after the age of 35-40 have all been found to have neuropathology consistent with a diagnosis of Alzheimer disease (eg, Malamud 1972; Mann 1988; Wisniewski et al. 1985). It is important to note the wording here. Current convention considers Alzheimer disease to be a 'clinico-pathological' entity, and diagnosis depends upon a history of dementia together with the characteristic pattern of neuropathology (The National Institute on Aging and Reagan Institute Working Group on Diagnostic Criteria for the Neuropathological Assessment of Alzheimer Disease 1997). Documentation of dementia for adults with Down syndrome is as yet quite problematic, as will be discussed in the next section, and therefore it is important to emphasize that all adults with Down syndrome, while at risk, do not in fact have Alzheimer disease.

Amyloid-ß deposits make up the predominant pathological change seen in the brains of adults with Down syndrome once they reach their 30s. Quantitatively, amyloid-ß load in brains is clearly elevated beyond levels typically seen in Alzheimer disease cases without Down syndrome, and some investigators have observed that amyloid-ß load is significantly associated with dementia in these patients (Cummings et al. 1996). Nevertheless, there is evidence that neurofibrillary pathology is also of major importance in the development of dementia (eg, Braak and Braak 1991, 1997), even within the Cummings et al. sample, and neurofibrillary pathology comparable in severity to their amyloid-ß pathology is not universal among adults with Down syndrome of middle age and older (eg, Wisniewski et al. 1985).

As mentioned earlier, amyloid-ß plaques vary in structure. Neuritic plaques are associated with disruption of neuron functioning but diffuse plaques, which do not contain significant fibrillar components, have as yet not been linked to any clear effect on surrounding cells (cf. Wisniewski and Silverman 1997). Wisniewski et al. (1994) reported that formation of diffuse rather than neuritic plaques characterizes the brains of nondemented adults with Down syndrome, and that they show some, but not all, of the brain pathology typical of Alzheimer disease. Another recent study has indicated distinctions between neurofibrillary pathology seen in Alzheimer disease and in ageing adults with Down syndrome (Muketova-Ladinska et al. 1995). Therefore, evidence is accumulating that the pathological changes that occur in Alzheimer disease and with ageing in adults with Down syndrome may not be quite the same.

Recognition of dementia among adults with Down syndrome

In their consensus statement, Small et al. (1997) discussed the importance of diagnosing dementia based upon significant decline from an individual's previous levels of performance or functioning. This is particularly true for adults with mental retardation and Down syndrome, all of whom will have lifelong impairments in cognitive and functional abilities (eg, American Association on Mental Retardation 1992). Unfortunately, all procedures that have been broadly disseminated to assess primary progressive dementias, including Alzheimer disease, were developed for use with nonretarded adults. Therefore, there are no 'standard' methods or criteria in place for diagnosis of dementia in adults with Down syndrome.

This lack of standards for diagnosis needs to be addressed for many reasons. First, estimates of prevalence of dementia can vary substantially depending upon criteria for case classification, even when well established assessment methods are available (Erkinjuntti et al. 1997). This imprecision creates clear difficulties for programme planners who need to be able to estimate case load and patterns of service need.

Second, there are many treatable conditions that can mimic the symptoms of dementia in adults with Down syndrome and other conditions resulting in mental retardation. These include reactions to psychoactive medications (Seltzer and Luchterhand 1994), depression (eg, Burt et al. 1995), hypothyroidism (eg, Prasher 1995), and any other chronic health condition or illness that could involve depressed performance as a component of atypical clinical presentation in adults lacking adequate expressive language skills. For older adults with Down syndrome, some care providers may be biased towards assuming that any indication of declining performance represents the onset of Alzheimer disease. There could be many occasions when Alzheimer disease will not in fact be the cause of declines of concern, and treatable conditions can only be identified through further diagnostic evaluations. Until procedures for differential diagnosis of adults with Down syndrome have achieved levels of precision comparable with those that now exist for adults without mental retardation, it is vital that a thorough evaluation be done for any person suspected of dementia. Treatment should then be provided for any condition or illness discovered, no matter how apparently tenuous the connection with dementia symptoms, because it is always possible that performance declines might be associated with illness, discomfort, sensory deficit, depression, and so on.

Establishing the absence of dementia among adults with Down syndrome

Evidence of frank dementia seems to be absent for many adults with Down syndrome, even once they reach ages at which the presence of neuropathology consistent with Alzheimer disease is a virtual certainty (see Silverman et al. 1998 for a recent review). Prevalence estimates vary considerably among the many studies of dementia in this population, and range from under 10 per cent to over 70 per cent (see Zigman et al. 1997). These substantial differences are no doubt due, at least in part, to variations in sampling procedures, criteria for case classification, and ages of participants. However, given the limits on our current abilities to diagnose Alzheimer dementia in adults with Down syndrome, arguments have been made that the early and subtle symptoms are simply being overlooked and true prevalence approaches 100 per cent. If neuropathology consistent with Alzheimer disease approaches universal presence, then a strong burden of proof must be imposed upon claims that dementia can be absent. This is especially important because of the far-reaching implications of such a disparity between neuropathology and clinical profiles. It would indicate that the clear amyloid-ß pathology virtually guaranteed to be present is not necessarily linked to clinical consequences, and in turn this would call into question predominant current models of Alzheimer disease pathogenesis.

While it is always difficult to demonstrate convincingly the absence of a condition, this can be done in the case of Alzheimer dementia, but only under the right set of circumstances. The clinical course and rate of progression of Alzheimer dementia have both been well described (eg, Reisberg et al. 1989). The characteristics of end stage disease are so dramatic that they cannot be overlooked, even in those adults with Down syndrome having relatively severe pre-existing cognitive and adaptive deficits. Therefore, because Alzheimer disease, if truly present, must produce unmistakable declines in status as it progresses, demonstrations of stable performance in older adults with Down syndrome over a period of several years would provide convincing verification that dementia need not in fact be present.

If the rate of clinical progression is comparable for adults with and without Down syndrome and significant Alzheimer disease neuropathology is present for adults with Down syndrome when they are 30-40 years of age, then dementia should be evident by the time they reach 50-55, taking into account the fact that early symptoms could be overlooked and only the obvious clinical involvement characteristic of more advanced disease would be reliably detected. To detect this dementia, longitudinal studies merely have to assess adults with Down syndrome in their 40s, 50s and 60s repeatedly over the course of several years to document declines in status. This has now been done by several groups (eg, Devenny et al 1996; Evenhuis 1990; Haxby and Shapiro 1992; Rasmussen and Sobsey 1994; Schupf et al. 1989; Vicari et al. 1994; Zigman et al. 1996), and we will summarize the results of two of these reports from our Institute.

Zigman et al. (1996) examined changes in adaptive behaviour among two very large groups of adults with mental retardation, one with Down syndrome and one without. Data were obtained from records of performance collected annually employing an adaptive behaviour scale included within a statewide database that had been in use throughout New York. Analyses determined the proportion of adults at any given age showing declines in adaptive behaviours over a multiyear period, and assumed that any person with Alzheimer disease would be among the declining subgroup. Of course, scales of adaptive behaviour were not originally designed to assess Alzheimer disease, per se, and declines could occur for any number of reasons in addition to dementia (eg, sensory loss, injury, chronic illness). Nevertheless, while false positive cases should be expected, there are no extraneous factors that should cause cases with Alzheimer disease to be overlooked once progression is sufficiently advanced. Therefore, given the time frames outlined earlier, close to 100 per cent prevalence of significant declines among adults with Down syndrome would be expected once they reached their mid-50s if Alzheimer disease were truly present.

No definitive criterion for 'significant' decline has yet been established for existing adaptive behaviour scales, and therefore Zigman et al. (1996) conducted several analyses employing classification criteria of decline that ranged from liberal to stringent. Fortunately, key findings converged across criteria, and indicated that adults with Down syndrome were no more likely to be declining than were adults with other forms of mental retardation up to the age of 50. Because other adults were not at risk for Alzheimer disease at these ages, this suggests that dementia was not characteristic of adults with Down syndrome at this stage of life (although occasional cases with dementia can occur). After age 50, the prevalence of decline for adults with Down syndrome increased relative to their peers with mental retardation due to other causes, but declines were far from universal even after 60 years of age. These analyses clearly demonstrated that some adults with Down syndrome were not showing declines in adaptive behaviour, and by extension were not demented, despite the Alzheimer neuropathology they had to have experienced for some 10 to 30 years.

Of course, it is possible to maintain that these measures of adaptive behaviours were not sensitive to the specific changes that characterize dementia. Indeed, it has to be conceded that these assessments were designed for purposes completely unrelated to the Zigman et al. (1996) application. Nevertheless, the conclusions as described seem valid given the extended time frame that was examined, but converging evidence based upon tasks designed more explicitly for the purpose of examining dementia would substantially strengthen the case being made here.

Fortunately, this evidence has been provided in a number of studies (cf. Silverman et al. 1998), of which Devenny et al. (1996) will serve as our example. They employed a battery of tests to examine domains of memory and cognition known to be affected during early stages of Alzheimer disease. Adults with Down syndrome and their peers without Down syndrome at similar ages and IQs, all of whom were nondemented and over 30 years of age when the study began, have been followed over the course of many years. (Devenny et al. reported findings up until 1995-96, but the study will continue at least until the year 2001.) While declines characteristic of Alzheimer disease among some participants were found, the performance profiles over the years indicated stability for most adults with Down syndrome over 50 years of age or slight declines indicative of 'normal' ageing. Overall, findings were consistent with Zigman et al. (1996) and similar studies of adaptive behaviour. In fact, this general pattern of results has now been described by many investigators employing a variety of assessment methods (see Silverman et al. 1998), and no longitudinal study has reported a prevalence of decline approaching 100 per cent for adults with Down syndrome in their 50s and 60s. Therefore, the conclusion that adults with Down syndrome can indeed be free of dementia in their 50s and 60s is now well justified.

Some adults with Down syndrome do succumb to Alzheimer disease, even before they reach 50 years of age, while others manage to avoid clinical involvement well into their 60s. If these individual differences can be understood, insights could lead to the development of strategies for treatment and prevention. In any event, the very fact that the consequences of Alzheimer disease can be delayed or avoided for some adults with Down syndrome suggests that factors in addition to the third copy of chromosome 21 exert significant influences on vulnerability. These factors need to identified and understood.

Down syndrome and the genetics of dementia

Part of the explanation for the individual differences in vulnerability to Alzheimer disease seen among adults with Down syndrome is likely to be related to genetic factors, some associated with genes located on chromosome 21 and some with genes on other chromosomes. As summarized earlier, multiple genetic loci have been linked to risk for Alzheimer disease and associated with its underlying mechanisms. For adults with Down syndrome, the gene coding for APP, located on chromosome 21, is obviously of major significance. People with Down syndrome appear to have an excess of amyloid-ß during their entire lives (eg, Teller et al. 1996), and over time this is bound to increase vulnerability to amyloid pathology. In fact, Prasher et al. (1998) just described a case study of a woman with Down syndrome who died at the age of 78 without ever having shown signs of dementia. The longevity of this woman and her 'successful' ageing appear to be related to the fact that she had partial trisomy, and the site of the APP gene was not present in triplicate. Most remarkably for an elderly person with Down syndrome, neuropathological changes consistent with Alzheimer disease were also not seen upon postmortem examination. This case study, though based on only one person, has very exciting implications for understanding the vulnerability of adults with Down syndrome, as well as for understanding the fundamental nature of Alzheimer pathogenesis.

Apo ϵ, located on chromosome 19, is an important determinant of risk for Alzheimer disease in the general population, and although there remains some controversy, it seems to operate similarly for adults with Down syndrome (eg, Schupf et al. 1996). Adults with Down syndrome with Apo ϵ-4 appear to be at increased risk, while those with Apo ϵ-2 are less likely to develop dementia. In fact, Schupf et al. found nobody with Apo ϵ-2 among their cases with physician diagnosed dementia, but as they stated, this subsample was neither large nor old enough to infer that having an Apo ϵ-2 allele provides complete protection. (Alzheimer cases with Apo ϵ-2 have occurred within the nonretarded population.)

Adults with Down syndrome exhibit many other physical changes usually taken as evidence of advancing age earlier in their lives than expected (Brown 1985). It seems probable that predisposition toward these other ageing changes is associated with overexpression of genes located on chromosome 21 distinct from the gene coding for APP, as we have discussed elsewhere (Wisniewski and Silverman 1996). These other genes have yet to be identified, but given that Alzheimer disease is so inextricably linked to ageing processes, the role(s) of these other genetic influences on lifespan development could be of great importance in determining individual risk. The products of these genes could exert their effects directly, or they could have indirect influences on the actions of proteins controlled by other genes (not necessarily located on chromosome 21), as well as with environmental factors.

Conclusions

As with any other aspect of lifespan development, mechanisms that are inherently complex, interactive and nonlinear are likely to be controlling changes in status over time as adults with Down syndrome age. This reality needs to be fully appreciated in attempts to account for the wide range of individual differences seen within this population. We already know that, despite its elevated risk for Alzheimer disease, trisomy 21 does not necessarily carry with it a predetermined and unavoidable destiny of progressive deterioration during middle age. The rapid advances currently being made in research laboratories throughout the world, targeting Down syndrome, Alzheimer disease, or both, are providing concrete indications that opportunities for 'successful' ageing can be enhanced in the future, even for the most vulnerable individuals. However, the key phenomena that need to be examined develop very slowly, sometimes over decades, and major investments in relevant research have only been made recently. The promise of current discoveries will only be realized through perseverance and patience.

Prospective studies that follow older adults from ages before dementia begins until symptoms are advanced can describe the natural history of dementia in the population of adults with Down syndrome, document the range of clinical profiles, and determine methods that are well suited for early diagnosis. In addition, these types of studies can relate vulnerability and characteristics of clinical progression to both genetic and nongenetic factors that determine risk. Eventually, understanding of the basic mechanisms involved in Alzheimer disease pathogenesis will be discovered, and effective methods to halt progression of the devastating destruction of neural systems eventually will become available. When that occurs, the effectiveness of intervention will be critically dependent upon early diagnosis. For adults with Down syndrome, effective methods for early recognition of dementia still need to be developed and factors that influence individual differences in risk need to be identified. These issues should be among the immediate targets of our current research agenda.

Acknowledgements

The authors gratefully acknowledge the support provided by New York State through its Office of Mental Retardation and Developmental Disabilities, as well as by Grants R01 AG09439, P01 AG11531 from the National Institute on Aging and P01 HD35897 from the National Institute of Child Health and Human Development.

References

Alzheimer A (1907) Über eine eigenartige Erkrankung der Hirnrinde. Allgemeine Zeitschrift für Psychiatrie und Psychisch-Gerichtliche Medizin 64 :146-8.

Aylward EH, Burt DB, Thorpe LU, Lai F, Dalton AJ (1997) Diagnosis of dementia in individuals with intellectual disability. Journal of Intellectual Disability Research 41: 152-64.

American Association on Mental Retardation (1992) Mental Retardation: Definition, Classification and Systems of Supports. Washington, DC: American Association on Mental Retardation.

Braak H, Braak E (1991) Neuropathological stageing of Alzheimer's changes. Acta Neuropathologica 82: 239-59.

Braak H, Braak E (1997) Frequency of stages of Alzheimer-related lesions in different age categories. Neurobiology of Aging 18: 351-7.

Braddock D, Hemp R, Parish S, Westrich J (1997) The State of the States in Developmental Disabilities. Washington, DC: American Association on Mental Retardation.

Brown WT (1985) Genetics of aging. In Janicki MP, Wisniewski HM (eds) Aging and Developmental Disabilities: Issues and Approaches. Baltimore, MD: Brookes. pp 185-94.

Burt D, Loveland K, Chen YW, Chuang A, Lewis K, Cherry L (1995) Aging in adults with Down syndrome: report from a longitudinal study. American Journal on Mental Retardation 100: 262-70.

Callahan C, Hendrie H, Tierney W (1995) Documentation and evaluation of cognitive impairment in elderly primary care patients. Annals of Internal Medicine 122: 422-9.

Corder E, Saunders A, Strittmatter W, Schmechel D, Gaskell P, Small G, Roses A, Haines S, Pericak-Vance M (1993) Gene dose of apolipoprotein E type 4 allele and the risk of Alzheimer's disease in late onset families. Science 261: 921-3.

Corder E, Saunders A, Risch N, Strittmatter W, Schmechel D, Gaskell P, Rimmler J, Locke P, Conneally P, Schmader K, Small G, Roses AL, Haines J, Pericak-Vance M (1994) Protective effect of apolipoprotein E type 2 alleles decreases the risk of late onset Alzheimer disease. Nature Genetics 7: 180-4.

Cummings B, Pike C, Shanakle R, Cotman C (1996) ß-amyloid deposition and other measures of neuropathology predict cognitive status in Alzheimer disease. Neurobiology of Aging 17: 921-33.

Devenny D, Silverman W, Hill AL, Jenkins E, Sersen E, Wisniewski K (1996) Normal aging in adults with Down syndrome: a longitudinal study. Journal of Intellectual Disability Research 40: 208-21.

Evans DA (1990) Estimated prevalence of Alzheimer disease in the United States. Milbank Quarterly 68: 267-89.

Erkinjuntti T, Ostbye T, Steenhuis R, Hachinski V (1997) The effect of different diagnostic criteria on the prevalence of dementia. New England Journal of Medicine 337: 1667-74.

Evenhuis H (1990) The natural history of dementia in Down's syndrome. Archives of Neurology 47: 263-7.

Folstein M, Folstein S, McHugh P (1975) 'Mini-Mental State': a practical method for grading the cognitive state of patients for the clinician. Journal of Psychiatric Research 12: 189-98.

Goate A, Chartier-Harlin M, Mullan M, Brown J, Crawford F, Fidani L, Giuffra L, Haynes A, Irving N, James L, Ment R, Newton P, Rooke K, Roques P, Talbot D, Pericak-Vance M, Roses A, Williamson R, Rossor M, Owen M, Hardy J (1991) Segregation of a missense mutation in the amyloid precursor protein gene with familial Alzheimer's disease. Nature 349: 704-6.

Hardy J, Higgins G (1992) Alzheimer's disease: the amyloid cascade hypothesis. Science 256: 184-5.

Haxby J, Shapiro M (1992) Longitudinal study of neuropsychological function in older adults with Down syndrome. In Nadel L, Epstein C (eds) Down Syndrome and Alzheimer's Disease. New York: Wiley-Liss. pp. 35-50.

Hook E (1981) Down's syndrome: frequency in human populations and factors pertinent to variation in rates. In De la Cruz F, Gerald P (eds) Trisomy 21 (Down's Syndrome). Baltimore, MD: University Park Press. pp. 3-67.

Larson E, Edwards J, O'Meara E, Nochlin D, Sumi S (1996) Neuropathologic diagnostic outcomes from a cohort of outpatients with suspected dementia. Journal of Gerontology 51: M313-M318.

Levy-Lehad E, Wasco W, Poorkaj P, Romano D, Oshima J, Pettingell W, Yu C, Jondro P, Schmidt S, Wang K, Crowley A, Fu YH, Guenette S, Galas D, Nemens E, Wijsman E, Bird T, Schellenberg G, Tanzi R (1995) Candidate gene for the chromosome 1 familial Alzheimer's disease locus. Science 269: 973-7.

Malamud N (1972) Neuropathology of organic brain syndrome associated with aging. In Gaitz CM (ed) Aging and the Brain. New York: Plenum. pp. 67-87.

Mann DMA (1988) Alzheimer's disease and Down's syndrome. Histopathology 13: 125-37.

Mirra S, Gearing M, Heyman A (1994) CERAD Guide to the Neuropathological Assessment of Alzheimer's Disease and other Dementias. Durham, NC: CERAD.

Muketova-Ladinska E, Harrington C, Roth M, Wischik C (1995) Distribution of tau protein in Downs's syndrome: quantitative differences from Alzheimer's disease. Developmental Brain Dysfunction 7: 311-29.

The National Institute on Aging and Reagan Institute Working Group on Diagnostic Criteria for the Neuropathological Assessment of Alzheimer's Disease (1997) Consensus recommendations for the postmortem diagnosis of Alzheimer's disease. Neurobiology of Aging 18, 54: 51-2.

Neurobiology of Aging (1997) Vol. 18 (No.S4) S1-S105.

Pericak-Vance M, Bass M, Yamaoka L, Gaskell P, Scott W, Terwedow H, Menold M, Conneally PM, Small G, Vance J, Saunders A, Roses A, Haines J (1997) Complete genomic screen in late-onset familial Alzheimer disease. Journal of the American Medical Association 278: 1237-41.

Prasher V (1995) Age-specific prevalence, thyroid dysfunction and depressive symptomatology in adults with Down syndrome and dementia. International Journal of Geriatric Psychiatry 10: 25-31.

Prasher V, Frarrer M, Kessling A, Fisher E, West R, Barber P, Butler A (1998) Molecular mapping of Alzheimer-type dementia in Down's syndrome. Annals of Neurology 43: 380-3.

Rasmussen DE, Sobsey D (1994) Age, adaptive behavior and Alzheimer disease in Down syndrome: Cross-sectional and longitudinal analyses. American Journal on Mental Retardation 99: 151-65.

Reisberg B, Ferris S, DeLeon M, Kluger A, Franssen E, Borenstein J, Alba R (1989) The stage specific temporal course of Alzheimer's disease: functional and behavioral concomitants based upon cross-sectional and longitudinal observation. In Iqbal K, Wisniewski HM, Winblad B (eds) Alzheimer's Disease and Related Disorders. New York: Alan R Liss. pp. 23-41.

Robakis N, Wisniewski H, Jenkins E, Devine-Gage E, Houck G, Yao X, Ramakrishna R, Wolfe G, Silverman W, Brown WT (1987) Chromosome 21q17 sublocalization of the gene encoding the beta-amyloid peptide in vessels and neuritic (senile) plaques of people with Alzheimer's disease and Down syndrome. Lancet 1: 384-5.

Rogaev E, Sherrington R, Rogaeva E, Levesque G, Ikeda M, Liang Y, Chi H, Lin C, Holman K, Tsuda T, Mar L, Sorbi S, Nacmais B, Piacentini S, Amaducci L, Chumakov I, Cohen D, Launfelt L, Fraser P, Rommens J, St George-Hyslop P (1995) Familial Alzheimer's disease in kindreds with missense mutations in a gene of chromosome 1 related to the Alzheimer's disease type 3 gene. Nature 376: 775-8.

Ryan D (1994) Misdiagnosis in dementia; Comparisons of diagnostic error rate and range of hospital investigation according to medical specialty. International Journal of Geriatric Psychiatry 9: 141-7.

Schupf N, Silverman WP, Sterling RC, Zigman WB (1989) Down syndrome, terminal illness and risk for dementia of the Alzheimer type. Brain Dysfunction 2: 181-8.

Schupf N, Kapell D, Lee JH, Zigman W, Canto B, Tycko B, Mayeux R (1996) Onset of dementia is associated with apolipoprotein E 4 in Down's syndrome. Annals of Neurology 40: 799-801.

Seltzer G, Luchterhand C (1994) Health and well-being of older persons with developmental disabilities: A clinical review In Seltzer M, Krauss M, Janicki M (eds) Life Course Perspectives on Adulthood and Old Age. Washington DC: American Association on Mental Retardation. pp. 109-42.

Sherrington R, Rogaev E, Liang Y, Rogaeva E, Levesque G, Ikeda M, Chi H, Lin C, Li G, Holman K, Tsuda T, Mar L, Foncin J-F, Bruni A, Montesi M, Sorbi S, Rainero I, Pinessi L, Nee L, Chumakov I, Pollen D, Pericak-Vance M, Tanzi R, Roses A, Fraser P,

Rommens J, St George-Hyslop P (1995) Cloning of a novel gene bearing missense mutations in early familial Alzheimer disease. Nature, 375: 754-60.

Silverman W, Zigman W, Kim H, Krinsky-McHale S, Wisniewski HM (1998) Aging and dementia among adults with mental retardation and Down syndrome. Topics in Geriatric Rehabilitation 13: 49-64.

Small G, Rabins P, Barry P, Buckholtz N, DeKosky S, Ferris S, Finkel S, Gwyther L, Khachaturian Z, Lebowitz B, McRae T, Morris J, Oakley F, Schneider L, Streim J, Sunderland T, Teri L, Tune L (1997) Diagnosis and treatment of Alzheimer's disease and related disorders. Consensus statement of the American Association for Geriatric Psychiatry, the Alzheimer's Association, and the American Geriatrics Society. Journal of the American Medical Association 278: 1363-71.

Strauss D, Eyman R (1996) Mortality of people with mental retardation in California with and without Down syndrome. American Journal on Mental Retardation 100: 643-53.

Strittmatter W, Saunders A, Schmechal D, Pericak-Vance M, Enghold J, Salvesen G, Roses A (1993). Apolipoprotein E: High affinity to ß-amyloid and increased frequency of type 4 allele in late-onset familial Alzheimer's disease Proceedings of the National Academy of Sciences USA 90: 1977-81.

Struwe F (1929) Histopathologisch untersuchungen über Entstehung und Wesen der senilen plaques. Zeitschrift für die Gesamte Neurologie und Psychiatrie 122: 291-307.

Teller J, Russo C, DeBusk L, Angelini G, Zaccheo D, Dagna-Bricarelli F, Scartezzini P, Bertolini S, Mann DMA, Tabaton M, Gambetti P (1996) Presence of soluble amyloid-ß peptide precedes amyloid plaque formation in Down's syndrome. Nature Medicine 2: 93-5.

Terry R, Katzman R (1983) Senile dementia of the Alzheimer type. Annals of Neurology 14: 497-506.

Vicari S, Nocentini U, Caltagirone C (1994) Neuropsychological diagnosis of aging in adults with Down syndrome. Developmental Brain Dysfunction 7: 340-8.

Visser F, Aldenkamp A, van Huffelen A, Kuilman M, Overweg J, van Wijk J (1997) Prospective study of the prevalence of Alzheimer-type dementia in institutionalized individuals with Down syndrome American Journal on Mental Retardation 101: 400-12.

WHO (1992) International statistical classification of diseases and related disorders. Tenth revision. Geneva: World Health Organization. pp. 312-14.

Wisniewski HM, Silverman W (1996) Alzheimer disease, neuropathology and dementia in Down syndrome. In Rondal JA, Nadel L, Perrera J (eds) Down Syndrome: Psychological, Psychobiological, and Socio-educational Perspectives. London: Whurr. pp. 43-52.

Wisniewski H, Silverman W (1997) Diagnostic criteria for the neuropathological assessment of Alzheimer's disease: current status and major issues. Neurobiology of Aging 18, S4: S43-S50.

Wisniewski H, Wegiel J, Kotula L (1996) Some neuropathological aspects of Alzheimer disease and its relevance to other disciplines. Journal of Neuropathology and Applied Neurobiology 22: 3-11.

Wisniewski HM, Wegiel J, Popovitch ER (1994) Age associated development of diffuse and thioflavin-S-positive plaques in Down syndrome. Developmental Brain Dysfunction 7: 330-9.

Wisniewski KE, Wisniewski HM, Wen GY (1985) Occurrence of neuropathological changes and dementia of Alzheimer's disease in Down syndrome. Annals of Neurology 17: 278-82.

Zigman WB, Schupf N, Sersen E, Silverman W (1996) Prevalence of dementia in adults with and without Down syndrome. American Journal on Mental Retardation 100: 403-12.

Zigman WB, Seltzer GB, Silverman W (1994) Behavioral and mental health changes associated with aging in adults with mental retardation with or without Down syndrome. In Seltzer MM, Krauss MW, Janicki MP (eds), Life Course Perspectives on Adulthood and Old Age. Washington, DC: American Association on Mental Retardation. pp. 67-94.

Zigman W, Schupf N, Haaveman M, Silverman W (1997) The epidemiology of Alzheimer disease in intellectual disability: results and recommendations from an international conference. Journal of Intellectual Disability Research 41: 76-80.

PART 6
GENETICS

Chapter 18
Towards the Identification of the Genes Involved in the Pathogenesis of Down Syndrome

PIERRE-MARIE SINET

Introduction

Chromosome 21, the smallest human chromosome (1.5 per cent of the genome), is around 50 Megabases of DNA in length and is supposed to contain between 500 and 1,000 genes. Its presence in three copies instead of two in cells of an individual is responsible for Down syndrome.

Due to the gene excess, the messenger RNA and proteins encoded by chromosome 21 genes are synthesized in larger amounts than normal, and this increase is usually proportional to the gene overdosage, that is by 50 per cent. This gene dosage effect has been shown for superoxide dismutase-1 (SOD1) (Sinet et al. 1974), α-interferon receptor (IFNAR) (Epstein et al. 1982; Gerdes et al. 1993), liver-type phosphofructokinase (PFKL) (Anneren et al. 1987), lymphocyte function-associated antigen (LFA1 or CD18 or ITGB2) (Taylor et al. 1988), chromosomal protein HMG14 (Pash et al. 1991), S-100 protein (Kato et al. 1991) and carbonyl reductase (CBR) (Lemieux et al. 1993) and is expected to occur for any gene on chromosome 21.

Down syndrome is the most frequent among birth defects, afflicting 1 in 700 liveborn infants. It is characterized by a complex phenotype, variable in its expression from one trisomy 21 patient to another, and associated modifications of the morphogenesis of the face, limbs, hands and feet, including visceral malformations (eg, heart, gut), impairment of physiological constants such as decreased muscle tone and hyperlaxity of the joints, features of accelerated ageing and a constant mental delay. With very few exceptions, the biological bases of these defects are not yet known.

The goal of biological research on Down syndrome is to find which gene(s) and protein(s) in excess contribute to the main features of this phenotype, and therefore, to understand the pathophysiological bases of the disease.

Genotype-phenotype analysis of patients with partial trisomy 21 led to the identification of chromosome 21 regions contributing to the pathogenesis of Down syndrome features

One step towards the identification of genes that could play a role in the pathogenesis of Down syndrome is the definition, as concisely as possible, of minimal regions on chromosome 21 involved in producing particular features of the phenotype (Epstein et al. 1991). This can be done by analyzing genotype-phenotype correlations in rare patients with partial trisomy 21. More than 15 years ago, clinical and karyotyping studies indicated that trisomy of the distal part of chromosome 21, namely band q22, was responsible for most of the clinical features of Down syndrome (Aula et al. 1973; Jenkins et al. 1983; Mattei et al. 1981; Sinet et al. 1976). In a review of most of the published observations of partial trisomies 21 at that time, it was concluded that the duplication of a fraction of 21q22, close to sub-band 21q22.2, had a critical role for the pathogenesis of Down syndrome (Park et al. 1987).

More recently, molecular analysis of patients with partial trisomy 21 has confirmed the proposition of a significant role for 21q22 in Down syndrome pathogenesis. Table 18.1 describes chromosome 21 and some regions contributing to various features of Down syndrome (Delabar et al. 1993; Korenberg et al. 1990, 1992, 1994; McCormick et al. 1989; Petersen et al. 1990; Rahmani et al. 1989). The duplication of the D21S55 region, located inside or close to subband 21q22.2, is associated with many of the clinical features characteristic of the syndrome, which suggests that genes within this region are important for the phenotypic expression of trisomy 21 (Delabar et al. 1993; Rahmani et al. 1989).

As indicated in Figure 18.1, genes outside the D21S55 region also contribute to various aspects of the phenotype (Korenberg et al. 1994). For example, APP (Amyloid Precursor Protein) and SOD1 genes play a role in the genesis of Alzheimer-like neuropathology and ageing features respectively. Moreover, several genes in excess may be required for generating some phenotypic features. This is particularly likely for complex phenotypic features such as mental retardation.

The study of patients with partial trisomy 21 needs to be extended by improving the phenotypic description at the clinical, psychological and biological levels, and by defining more precisely at the molecular level the exact extent and location of the chromosome 21 segments present in triplicate. These data will definitely increase in our understanding of Down syndrome.

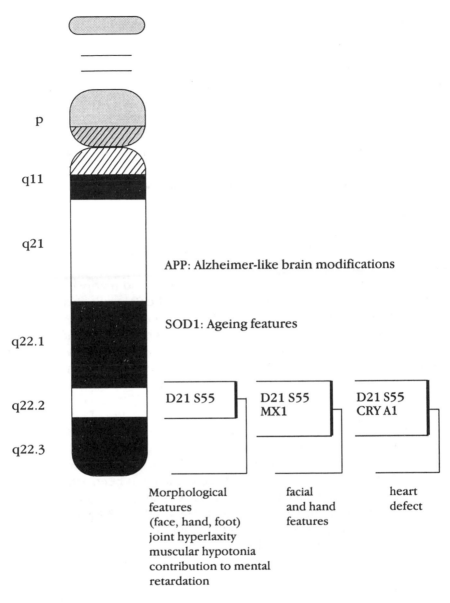

APP: Amyloid precursor protein gene
SOD1: Superoxide dismutase-1 gene
D21S55: DNA marker
MX1: Myxovirus (influenza) resistance 1 gene
CRYA1: Crystallin, alpha polypeptide 1 gene

Figure 18.1 Two genes (APP and SOD1) and three regions of chromosome 21 contributing to phenotypic features of Down syndrome.

Identification and mapping of genes on chromosome 21 is progressing exponentially

A search for the genes present on chromosome 21 and particularly in the regions involved in phenotypic features of Down syndrome has been undertaken, using various techniques such as exon-trapping (Chen et al. 1996; Dahmane et al. 1998; Guimera et al. 1997; Lucente et al. 1995; Tassone et al. 1995; Yaspo et al. 1995), cDNA selection (Cheng et al. 1994; Dahmane et al. 1998; Ohira et al. 1997; Peterson et al. 1994) expressed-sequence tag (EST) collection (Chiang et al. 1995), cDNA amplification (Kurnit et al. 1995), and cDNA screening (Ohira et al. 1997). Furthermore, a multicentre programme for the DNA sequencing of chromosome 21 is currently underway (http://chr21.rz-berlin.mpg.de/rec22.html) and the DNA sequence of almost all of the chromosome is expected to be available by the end of 2002, which will contribute to establishing the repertoire of genes on chromosome 21.

So far, around 80 genes have been identified and mapped on chromosome 21, the biological role of which is either clearly known or only deducible (or imaginable) from structural similarities to genes previously described in humans or other organisms. Besides these 'known' genes, there are pieces of many other genes (exons or cDNAs) that have been identified but have not yet been named, either because information about their DNA sequence is still too limited or because they do not have sequence similarity to known genes.

It would be too fastidious to give an exhaustive list of all the 'known' genes currently mapped on chromosome 21. Instead, I will illustrate the progress in this field by summarizing our current knowledge of the D21S55 region. The physical mapping and cloning of this region, which spans 2.5 Mb DNA between genes CBR and ERG, has been achieved (Crété et al. 1993; Dufresne-Zacharia et al. 1994; Gosset et al. 1995; Ohira et al. 1996a; Osoegawa et al. 1996; Patil et al. 1994). About 30 genes have been identified and mapped (Dahmane et al. 1998; Guimera et al. 1997; Ohira et al. 1997), among which only eight are known genes (see Table 18.1). The biological function of only three of these known genes, CAF1P60, HCS and GIRK2, has been established.

CAF1P60 (Blouin et al. 1996a; Katsanis and Fisher 1996) encodes the p60 subunit of chromatin assembly factor I (CAFI) (Kaufman et al. 1995). CAFI is a trimeric protein responsible for assembling the nucleosome by chaperoning histones to form the histone octamer that binds to DNA. The overexpression of CAF1P60 in trisomy 21 may disrupt the stoichiometry of the CAFI trimer, changing chromatin configuration and affecting gene expression.

HCS encodes the holocarboxylase synthetase enzyme that catalyzes biotin incorporation into several carboxylases involved in fatty acid synthesis, gluconeogenesis and amino acid catabolism (Leon-Del-Rio et al. 1995; Suzuki et al. 1994). Increased expression of HCS in Down syndrome may affect essential metabolic pathways (Blouin et al. 1996b).

Table 18.1 'Known' genes in the D21S55 region of chromosome 21

Gene	Sequence similarity to	Known or supposed function
KIAA0136	cDNA fom human myeloid cell line	Signal transduction
CAF1P60 P60 subunit of chromatin assembly factor-1		DNA replication, transcription and repair
SIM2 Single minded-2	Drosophila single minded	bHLH transcription factor, brain neurogenesis, cranio-facial morphogenesis
HCS Holocarboxylase synthetase		Biotin incorporation into carboxylases
TPRD gene containing a Tetratricopeptide repeat domain in the Down syndrome region	• Phosphatase (rat) • heat shock protein (yeast) • transformation sensitive protein (human)	Cell-division cycle, RNA synthesis
MNB minibrain	Drosophila minibrain rat dyrk yeast yak1	Protein kinase, cell cycle, cell proliferation, neurogenesis
GIRK2 (or KIR 3.2 or KCNJ6)	G protein-activated inward rectifier potassium channel	Neuronal excitability
KIR4.2 IRKK (or KCNJ15)	Inward rectifier potassium channel	Potassium cell permeability, neuronal excitability

GIRK2 encodes an inwardly rectifying potassium channel which contributes to the maintenance of resting potential and controls the excitability of cells. GIRK2 (Ferrer et al. 1995; Patil et al. 1995; Sakura et al. 1995; Tsaur et al. 1995) is expressed in the developing cerebellum of mice, and in many areas of the adult mouse brain including the cerebellum granule cells. It is also expressed in testes and pancreas (Kobayashi et al. 1995; Mjaatvedt at al. 1995; Patil et al. 1995). Its expression has also been detected in the adult human brain (Tanizawa et al. 1996). A point mutation in the pore-forming region of GIRK2 is responsible for the weaver pheno-type in mouse (Mjaatvedt et al. 1995; Patil et al. 1995). GIRK2-deficient mice develop spontaneous seizures and are more susceptible to drug-induced seizures, indicating that GIRK2 mediates neuronal excitability in vivo (Signorini et al. 1997).

Three of the other known genes may be involved in the development or physiology of the central nervous system. They may, therefore, be candidates for involvement in the mental retardation characteristic of Down syndrome.

Two genes, SIM2 (Chen et al. 1995; Chrast et al. 1997; Dahmane et al. 1995) encoding a basic helix-loop-helix transcription factor (Nambu et al. 1991; Thomas et al. 1988), and MNB (Guimera et al. 1996; Patil et al. 1995; Shindoh et al. 1996; Song et al. 1996) encoding a serine-threonine protein kinase (Tejedor et al. 1995) were originally identified in Drosophila and both are involved in the development of the central nervous system. These two genes are also expressed at early stages of brain development in mammals. In human, rat (Dahmane et al. 1995) and mouse (Fan et al. 1996; Moffet et al. 1996; Yamaki et al. 1996), the foetal expression pattern of SIM2 strongly suggests that it plays a central role in neurogenesis and early regionalization of the diencephalon. SIM2 is also expressed in cranio-facial structures, axial skeleton and muscle, and may, therefore, also be involved in hypotonia and the generation of several of the morphological features characteristic of trisomy 21. MNB is expressed in brain gray matter, the spinal cord and the retina during development in mouse (Song et al. 1996). In adult mice, it is expressed in several areas of the central nervous system (Guimera et al. 1996). Mice transgenic for a 180 kb YAC containing the MNB gene have been reported to suffer from spatial learning and memory deficits, suggesting that overexpression of MNB may contribute to the learning defects associated with Down syndrome (Smith et al. 1997).

KIR4.2 (Gosset et al. 1997; Ohira et al. 1997) encodes an inwardly rectifying potassium channel of the same family as GIRK2. It is expressed in developing kidney and lung tissues in humans and in several adult tissues including brain (Gosset et al. 1997). Thus, it may also be involved in brain physiology.

Finally, the two genes KIAA 0136 (Nagase et al. 1995) and TPRD (Ohira 1996b) contain sequence domains similar to those found in genes proteins involved in signal transduction or the control of cell cycle and RNA synthesis encoding.

Future research will be devoted to the discovery of the biological function of the chromosome 21 genes and to the assessment of their role in Down syndrome

As in the rest of chromosome 21, only a minority of genes of the D21S55 region (three of 30 genes, CAF1P60, HCS and GIRK2) have a clearly established biological function. For genes with known functions, it is possible to make hypotheses with regard to their potential pathogenic role in Down syndrome, and in order to test these hypotheses transgenic mice are suitable research tools. For example, data on transgenic mice for SOD1 are consistent with the concept that excess SOD1 contributes to a constitutive oxidative stress (Sinet 1982) leading to some of the ageing manifestations such as early thymus involution (Nabarra et al. 1996; Peled-Kamar et al. 1995) and abnormal neuromuscular junction (Avraham et al. 1988). Some lines of APP transgenic mice develop brain amyloid deposits and age-related learning deficits (Kammesheidt et al. 1992; Moran et al. 1995; Quon et al. 1991) indicating that APP overexpression plays a role in the constant occurrence of middle-age onset brain lesions that resemble those of Alzheimer disease. Mice transgenic for other genes such as ETS2 (Sumarsono et al. 1996), HMG14 (Bustin et al. 1995) and S100 (Reeves et al. 1994) have been reported with phenotypic features reminiscent of trisomy 21. Needless to say, systematically testing the phenotypic effects of every single gene would be extremely time consuming. More global approaches for producing particular phenotypic features are being carried out (see the chapter in this book by CJ Epstein) using partial trisomy 16 mice (part of the mouse chromosome 16 is homologous to almost all of human chromosome 21) or mice transgenic for multigenic DNA fragments (YAC, BAC, PAC). Finding a phenotypic feature reminiscent of Down syndrome will guarantee that interesting genes have been introduced into these mice and it will be worthwhile identifying it in them.

For five genes of the D21S55 region, KIAA0136, SIM2, TPRD, MNB and KIR4.2, firm hypotheses about function exist, based on sequence similarities with known genes and on experimental data in other organisms. These functional hypotheses need to be experimentally tested using modern biotechnology tools.

For a large majority of genes (around 2/3), sequence data are insufficient to propose any functional hypothesis. Expression during development and adult life in mouse and human tissues is required as the first step in functional studies of these genes.

Thus, as the identification of genes is being completed, a new and interesting period is opening: that of the functional studies of genes, and of assessment of their responsibility for the multiple facets of Down syndrome.

Acknowledgements

I would like to express my gratitude to the following colleagues for their contribution to the work presented in this chapter: V Abramowski, G Ait Ghezala, JL Blouin, M Casanova, I Céballos-Picot, Z Chamoun, Z Chettouh, N Créau, N Crété, N Dahmane, JM Delabar, MC Dufresne-Zacharia, E Fayet, S Gassanova-Maugenre, P Gosset, J London, C Lopes, C Maunoury, A

Nicole, D Paris, N Rabatel, Z Rahmani, K Toyama, C Vayssettes, ML Yaspo, and to MC Chasset for secretarial expertise.

Supported financially by Centre National de la Recherche Scientifique; Ministère de l'Education Nationale, de la Recherche et de la Technologie, EC Grants CT93-GENE0015 and BMH4-CT96-0554, Association Française contre les Myopathies; Université Paris V and Faculté de Médecine Necker-Enfants Malades.

References

Annerèn G, Korenberg JR, Epstein C (1987) Phosphofructokinase activity in fibroblasts aneuploid for chromosome 21. Human Genetics 76: 63-5.

Aula P, Leisti J, von Koskull H (1973) Partial trisomy 21. Clinical Genetics 4: 241-51.

Avraham KB, Schickler M, Sapoznikov D, Yarom R, Groner Y (1988) Down's syndrome: abnormal neuromuscular junction in tongue of transgenic mice with elevated levels of human Cu/Zn superoxide dismutase. Cell 54: 823-9.

Blouin JL, Duriaux-Sail G, Chen H, Gos A, Morris MA, Rossier C, Antonarakis SE (1996a) Mapping of the gene for the p60 subunit of the human chromatin assembly factor (CAF1A) to the Down syndrome region of chromosome 21. Genomics 33: 309-12.

Blouin JL, Duriaux-Saïl G, Antonarakis SE (1996b) Mapping of the human holocarboxylase synthetase (HCS) to the Down syndrome critical region of chromosome 21q22. Annals of Genetics 39: 185-8.

Bustin M, Alfonso PJ, Pash JM, Ward JM, Gearhart JD, Reeves RH (1995) Characterization of transgenic mice with an increased content of chromosomal protein HMG-14 in their chromatin. DNA Cell Biology 14, 997-1005.

Chen H, Chrast R, Rossier C, Gos A, Antonarakis SE, Kudoh J, Yamaki A, Shindoh N, Maeda H, Minoshima S, Shimizu N (1995) Single-minded and Down syndrome. Nature Genetics 10: 9-10.

Chen H, Chrast R, Rossier C, Morris M, Lalioti M, Antonarakis S (1996) Cloning of 559 potential exons of genes of human chromosome 21 by exon trapping. Genome Research 6: 747-60.

Cheng JF, Boyartchuk V, Zhu Y (1994) Isolation and mapping of human chromosome 21 cDNA: Progress in constructing a chromosome 21 expression map. Genomics 23: 75-84.

Chiang PW, Dzida G, Grumet J, Cheng JF, Song WJ, Crombez E, Van Keuren ML, Kurnit DM (1995) Expressed sequence tags from the long arm of human chromosome 21. Genomics 29: 383-9.

Chrast R, Scott HS, Chen H, Kudoh J, Rossier C, Minoshima S, Wang Y, Shimizu N, Antonarakis SE (1997) Cloning of two human homologs of the drosophila single-minded gene SIM1 on chromosome 6q and SIM2 on 21q within the Down syndrome chromosomal region. Genome Research 7: 615-24.

Crété N, Gosset P, Théophile D, Duterque-Coquillaud M, Blouin JL, Vayssette C, Sinet PM, Créau-Goldberg N (1993) Mapping the Down syndrome chromosomal region (DCR): establishment of a YAC contig spanning 1.2 Megabases. European Journal of Human Genetics 1: 51-63.

Dahmane N, Charron G, Lopes C, Yaspo ML, Maunoury C, Decorte L, Sinet PM, Bloch B, Delabar JM (1995) Down syndrome critical region contains a gene homologous to Drosophila sim expressed during rat and human central nervous system development. Proceedings of the National Academy of Science USA 92: 9191-5.

Dahmane N, Ghezala GA, Gosset P, Chamoun Z, Dufresne-Zacharia MC, Lopes C, Rabatel N, Gassanova-Maugenre S, Chettouh Z, Abramowski V, Fayet E, Yaspo ML, Korn B, Blouin JL, Lehrach H, Poutska A, Antonarakis SE, Sinet PM, Créau N, Delabar JM (1998) Transcriptional Map of the 2.5-Mb CBR-ERG Region of Chromosome 21 Involved in Down Syndrome. Genomics 48: 12-23.

Delabar JM, Théophile D, Rahmani Z, Chettouh Z, Blouin JL, Prieur M, Noel B, Sinet PM(1993) Molecular mapping of 24 features of Down syndrome on chromosome 21. European Journal of Human Genetics 1: 114-24.

Dufresne-Zacharia MC, Dahmane N, Théophile D, Orti R, Chettouh Z, Sinet PM, Delabar JM (1994) 3.6 Megabase genomic and YAC physical map of the Down syndrome region on chromosome 21. Genomics 19: 462-469.

Epstein CJ, McManus NH, Epstein LB, Branca AA, d'Allessandro SB, Baglioni C (1982) Direct evidence that the gene product of the human chromosome 21 locus, IFRC, is the interferon a receptor. Biochemistry and Biophysics Research 107, 1060-6.

Epstein CJ, Korenberg JR, Anneren G, Antonarakis SE, Aymé S, Courchesne E, Epstein LB, Fowler A, Groner Y, Huret JL, Kemper TL, Lott IR, Lubin BH, Magenis E, Opitz JM, Patterson D, Priest JH, Pueschel SM, Rapoport SI, Sinet PM, Tanzi RE, de la Cruz F (1991) Protocols to establish genotype-phenotype correlations in Down syndrome. American Journal of Human Genetics 49: 207-35.

Fan C-M, Kuwana E, Bulfone A, Fletcher CF, Copeland NG, Jenkins NA, Crews S, Martinez S, Puelles L, Rubinstein JLR, Tessier-Lavigne M (1996) Expression patterns of two murine homologs of Drosophila single-minded suggest possible roles in embryonic patterning and in the pathogenesis of Down syndrome. Molecular Cell Neurosciences 7: 1-16.

Ferrer J, Nichols CG, Makhina EN, Salkoff L, Bernstein J, Gerhard D, Wasson J, Ramanadham S, Permutt A (1995) Pancreatic islet cells express a family of inwardly rectifying K^+ channel subunits which interact to form G-protein-activated channels. Journal of Biological Chemistry 270: 26086-91.

Gerdes AM, Horder M, Petersen PH, Bonnevie-Nielsen V (1993) Effect of increased gene dosage expression on the α-interferon receptors in Down's syndrome. Biochemistry and Biophysics Acta. 1181: 135-40.

Gosset P, Crété N, Ait Ghezala G, Théophile D, Van Broeckhoven, Vayssettes C, Sinet PM, Créau N (1995) A high-resolution map of 1.6 Mb in the Down syndrome region: a new map between D21S55 and ETS2. Mamm. Genome 6: 127-30.

Gosset P, Ait Ghezala G, Korn B, Yaspo M-L, Poutska A, Lehrach H, Sinet P-M, Créau N (1997) A new inwardly rectifier potassium channel localized on chromosome 21 in the Down syndrome chromosome region 1 (DCR1). Genomics 44: 237-41.

Guimera J, Casas C, Pucharcos C, Solans A, Domènech A, Planas AM, Ashley J, Lovett M, Estivill X, Pritchard MA (1996) A human homologue of Drosophila minibrain (MNB) is expressed in the neuronal regions affected in Down syndrome and maps to the critical region. Human Molecular Genetics. 5: 1305-10.

Guimera J, Pucharcos C, Domènech A, Casas C, Solans A, Gallardo T, Ashley J, Lovett M, Estivill X, Pritchard M (1997) Cosmid contig and transcriptional map of three regions of human chromosome 21q22: Identification of 37 novel transcripts by direct selection. Genomics 45: 59-67.

Jenkins EC, Duncan CJ, Wright CE, Gordano FM, Wilbur L, Wisniewski K, Sklower SL, French JH, Jones C, Brown WT (1983) A typical Down syndrome and partial trisomy 21. Clinical Genetics 24: 97-102.

Kammesheidt A, Boyce FM, Spanoyannis AF, Cummings BJ, Ortegon M, Cotman C, Vaught JL, Neve RL (1992) Deposition of ß/A4 immunoreactivity and neuronal pathology in transgenic mice expressing the carboxy-terminal fragment of the

Alzheimer amyloid precursor in the brain. Proceedings of the National Academy of Science USA 89: 10857-61.

Kato K, Suzuki N, Kurobe K, Okajima N, Ogasawara M, Nagaya M, Yamanaka T (1991) Enhancement of S-100 beta protein in blood of patients with Down's syndrome. Journal of Molecular Neuroscience 2:109-13.

Katsanis N, Fisher EMC (1996) The gene encoding the p60 subunit of chromatin assembly factor I (CAF1P60) maps to human chromosome 21q22.2, a region associated with some of the major features of Down syndrome. Human Genetics 98: 497-9.

Kaufman PD, Kobayashi R, Kessler N, Stillman B (1995) The p150 and p60 subunits of chromatin assembly factor I: a molecular link between newly synthesized histones and DNA replication. Cell 81: 1105-14.

Kobayashi T, Ikeda K, Ichikawa T, Abe S, Togashi S, Kumanishi T (1995) Molecular cloning of a mouse G-protein-activated K+ channel (mGirk1) and distinct distributions of three Girk (Girk1, 2 and 3) mRNAs in mouse brain. Biochemistry and Biophysics Research 208: 1166-73.

Korenberg JR, Kawashima H, Pulst SM, Ikeuchi T, Ogasawara N, Yamamoto K, Schonberg SA, West R, Allen L, Magenis E, Ikawa K, Taniguchi N, Epstein CJ (1990) Molecular definition of a region of chromosome 21 that causes features of the Down syndrome phenotype. American Journal of Human Genetics 47: 236-46.

Korenberg JR, Bradley C, Disteche CM (1992) Down syndrome: Molecular mapping of the congenital heart disease and duodenal stenosis. American Journal of Human Genetics 50: 294-302.

Korenberg JR, Chen XN, Schipper R, Sun Z, Gonsky R, Gerwehr S, Carpenter N, Daumer C, Dignan P, Disteche C (1994) Down syndrome phenotypes: the consequences of chromosomal imbalance. Proceedings of the National Academy of Science USA 91: 4997-5001.

Kurnit DM, Cheng JF, Zhu Y, Van Keuren ML, Jiang Y, Pan Y-Z, Whitley K, Crombez E (1995) Transcription patterns of sequences on human chromosome 21. Cytogenetical Cell Genetics 71: 203-6.

Lemieux N, Malfoy B, Forrest GL (1993) Human carbonyl reductase (CBR) localized to band 21q22.1 by high resolution fluorescence in situ hybridization displays gene dosage effects in trisomy 21 cells. Genomics 15: 169-72.

Leon-Del-Rio A, Leclerc D, Akerman B, Wakamatsu N, Gravel RA (1995) Isolation of a cDNA encoding human holocarboxylase synthetase by functional complementation of a biotin auxotroph of Escherichia coli. Proceedings of the National Academy of Science USA 92: 4626-30.

Lucente D, Chen HM, Shea D, Samec SN, Rutter M, Chrast R, Rossier C, Buckler A, Antonarakis SE, McCormick MK (1995) Localization of 102 exons to a 2.5 Mb region involved in Down Syndrome. Human Molecular Genetics 4: 1305-11.

Mattei JF, Mattei G, Baeteman MA, Giraud F (1981) Trisomy 21 for the region 21q22.3: identification by high resolution R-banding patterns. Human Genetics 56: 409-11.

McCormick MK, Schinzel A, Petersen MB, Stetten G, Driscoll DJ, Cantu ES, Tranebjaerg L, Mikkelsen M, Watkins PC, Antonarakis SE (1989) Molecular genetic approach to the characterization of the 'Down syndrome Region' of chromosome 21.Genomics 5: 325-31.

Mjaatvedt AE, Cabin DE, Cole SE, Long LJ, Breitwieser GE, Reeves RH (1995) Assessment of a mutation in the H5 domain of Girk2 as a candidate for the weaver mutation. Genome Research 5: 453-63.

Moffet P, Dayo M, Reece M, McCormick MK, Pelletier J (1996) Characterization of msim, a murine homologue of the drosophila sim transcription factor. Genomics 35: 144-55.

Moran PM, Higgins LS, Cordell B, Moser PC (1995) Age-related learning deficits in transgenic mice expressing the 751-amino acid isoform of human ß-amyloid precuror protein. Proceedings of the National Academy of Science USA 92: 5341-5.

Nabarra B, Casanova M, Paris D, Nicole A, Toyama K, Sinet PM, Ceballos I, London J (1996) Trangenic mice overexpressing the human Cu/An SOD gene: ultrastructural studies of a premature thymic involution model of Down's syndrome (Trisomy 21). Laboratory Investigations 74: 3, 617.

Nagase T, Seki N, Tanaka A, Ishikawa K, Nomura N (1995) Prediction of the coding sequences of unidentified human genes.IV. The coding sequences of 40 new genes (KIAA0121-KIAA0160) deduced by analysis of cDNA clones from human cell line KG-1. DNA Research 2: 167-74.

Nambu JR, Lewis JO, Wharton KA, Crews ST (1991) The Drosophila single-minded gene encodes a helix-loop-helix protein that acts as a master regulator of CNS midline development. Cell, 67, 1157-67.

Ohira M, Ichikawa H, Suzuki E, Iwaki M, Suzuki K, Saito-Ohara F, Ikeuchi T, Chumakov I, Tanahashi H, Tashiro K, Sakaki Y, Ohki M (1996a) A 1.6 Mb P1 based physical map of the Down syndrome region on chromosome 21. Genomics 33, 65-74.

Ohira M, Ootsuyama A, Suzuki E, Ichikawa H, Seki N, Nagase T, Nomura N, Ohki M (1996b) Identification of a novel gene containing the tetratricopeptide repeat domain from the Down syndrome region of chromosome 21. DNA Research 3: 9-16.

Ohira M, Seki N, Nagase T, Suzuki E, Nomura N, Ohara O, Hattori M, Sakaki Y, Eki T, Murakami Y, Saito T, Ichikawa H, Ohki M (1997) Gene identification in 1.6 Mb region of the Down syndrome region on chromosome 21. Genome Research 7: 47-58.

Osoegawa K, Susukida R, Okano S, Kudoh J, Minoshima S, Shimizu N, De Jong PJ, Groet J, Ives J, Lehrach H, Nizetic D, Soeda E (1996) An integrated map with cosmid/PAC contigs of a 4-Mb Down syndrome critical region. Genomics 32: 375-87 .

Park JP, Wurster-Hill DH, Andrews PA, Cooley WC, Graham JM (1987) Free proximal trisomie 21 without the Down syndrome. Clinical Genetics 27: 128-44.

Pash J, Smithgall T, Bustin M (1991) Chromosomal protein HMG-14 overexpressed in Down syndrome. Experimental Cell Research 193: 232-5.

Patil N, Peterson A, Rothman A, de Jong PJ, Myers RM, Cox DR (1994) A high-resolution physical map of 2.5 Mbp of the Down syndrome region on chromosome 21. Human Molecular Genetics 3: 1811-17.

Patil N, Cox RC, Bhat D, Faham M, Myers RM, Peterson AS (1995) A potassium channel mutation in weaver mice implicates membrane excitability in granule cell differentiation. Nature Genetics 11: 126-9.

Peled-Kamar M, Lotem J, Okon E, Sachs L, Groner Y (1995) Thymic abnormalities and enhanced apoptosis of thymocytes and bone marrow cells in transgenic mice overexpressing Cu/Zn superoxide dismutase: implications for Down syndrome. The EMBO Journal 14, 20: 4985-93.

Petersen MB, Tranebjaerg L, McCormick MK, Michelsen N, Mikkelsen M, Antonarakis SE(1990) Clinical, cytogenetic and molecular genetic; characterization of two unrelated patients with different duplications of 21q. American Journal of Medical Genetics 7 (supplement): 105-9.

Peterson A, Patil N, Robbins C, Wang L, Cox DR, Myers RM (1994) A transcript map of the Down syndrome critical region on chromosome 21. Human Molecular Genetics 3: 1735-42.

Quon D, Wang Y, Catalano R, Marian Scardina J, Murakami K, Cordell B (1991) Formation of ß-amyloid protein deposits in brains of transgenic mice. Nature 352: 239-41.

Rahmani Z, Blouin JL, Créau-Goldberg N, Watkins PC, Mattei JF, Poissonier M, Prieur M, Chettouh Z, Nicole A, Aurias A, Sinet PM, Delabar JM (1989) Critical role of the D21S55 region on chromosome 21 in the pathogenesis of Down syndrome. Proceedings of the National Academy of Science USA 86: 5958-62.

Reeves RH, Yao J, Crowley MR, Buck S, Zhang X, Yarowsky P, Gearhart JD, Hilt DC (1994) Astrocytosis and axonal proliferation in the hippocampus of S100b transgenic mice. Proceedings of the National Academy of Science USA 91, 5359-63.

Sakura H, Bond C, Warren-Perry M, Horsley S, Kearney L, Tucker S, Adelman J, Turner R, Ashcroft FM (1995) Characterization and variation of a human inwardly-rectifying K-channel gene (KCNJ6): a putative ATP-sensitive K-channel subunit. FEBS Letter 367: 193-7.

Shindoh N, Kudoh J, Maeda H, Yamaki A, Minoshima S, Shimizu Y, Shimizu N (1996) Cloning of a human homolog of the Drosophila minibrain/ rat Dyrk gene from 'the Down syndrome critical region' of chromosome 21. Biochemistry and Biophysics Research 225: 92-9.

Signorini S, Joyce Liao Y, Duncan SA, Jan LY, Stoffel M (1997) Normal cerebellar development but susceptibility to seizures in mice lacking G protein-coupled, inwardly rectifying K$^+$ channel GIRK2. Proceedings of the National Academy of Science USA 94: 923-7.

Sinet PM (1982) Metabolism of oxygen derivatives in Down's syndrome. Annals of the New York Academy of Science 386:82-94.

Sinet PM, Allard D, Lejeune J, Jérome H (1974) Augmentation d'activité de la superoxyde dismutase érythrocytaire dans la trisomie pour le chromosome 21. Proceedings of the Academy of Science, Paris 278: 3267-70.

Sinet PM, Couturier J, Dutrillaux B, Poissonnier M, Raoul O, Rethoré MO, Allard D, Lejeune J, Jérome H (1976) Trisomie 21 et superoxyde dismutase (IPOA). Tentative de localisation sur la sous-bande 21q22.1. Experimental Cell Research 97: 47-55.

Smith DJ, Stevens ME, Sudanagunta SP, Bronson RT, Makhinson M, Watabe AM, O'Dell TJ, Fung J, Weier H-UG, Cheng J-F, Rubin EM (1997) Functional screening of 2Mb of human chromosome 21q22.2 in transgenic mice implicates minibrain in learning defects associated with Down syndrome. Nature Genetics 16: 28-36.

Song WJ, Sternberg LR, Kasten-Sportès C, Van Keuren ML, Chung SH, Slack AC, Miller DE, Glover TW, Chiang PW, Lou L, Kurnit DM (1996) Isolation of human and murine homologues of the Drosophila minibrain gene: human homologue maps to 21q22.2 in the Down syndrome 'critical region'. Genomics 38: 331-9.

Sumarsono SH, Wilson TJ, Tymms MJ, Venter DJ, Corrick CM, Kola R, Lahoud MH, Papas TS, Seth A, Kola I (1996) Down's syndrome-like skeletal abnormalities in Ets2 transgenic mice. Nature 379: 534-7.

Suzuki Y, Aoki Y, Ishida Y, Chiba Y, Iwamatsu A, Kishino T, Niikawa N, Matsubara Y, Narisawa K (1994) Isolation and characterization of mutations in the human holocarboxylase synthetase cDNA. Nature Genetics 8: 122-8.

Tanizawa Y, Matsubara A, Ueda K, Katagiri H, Kuwano A, Ferrer J, Permutt MA, Oka Y (1996) A human pancreatic islet inwardly rectifying potassium channel: cDNA cloning, determination of the genomic structure and genetic variations in Japanese NIDDM patients. Diabetologia 39: 447-52.

Tassone F, Xu H, Burkin H, Weissman S, Gardiner K (1995) cDNA selection from 10 Mb of chromosome 21 DNA: Efficiency in transcriptional mapping and reflections on genome organization. Human Molecular Genetics 4: 1509-18.

Taylor GM, Williams A, D'Souza SW, Fergusson WD, Donnai D, Fennell J, Harris R (1988) The expression of CD 18 is increased on trisomy 21 (Down syndrome) lymphoblastoid cells. Clinical Experimental Immunology 71: 324-8.

Tejedor F, Zhu XR, Kaltenbach E, Ackermann A, Baumann A, Canal I, Heisenberg M, Fischbach F, Pongs O (1995) Minibrain: a new protein kinase family involved in postembryonic neurogenesis in Drosophila. Neuron 14: 287-301.

Thomas JB, Crews ST, Goodman CS (1988) Molecular genetics of the single-minded locus: a gene involved in the development of the drosophila nervous system. Cell 52: 133-41.

Tsaur ML, Menzel T, Lai FP, Espinosa III R, Concannon P, Spielman RS, Hanis CL, Cox NJ, Le Beau MM, German MS, Jan LY, Bell GI, Stoffel M (1995) Isolation of a cDNA clone encoding a KATP channel-like protein expressed in insulin-secreting cells, localization of the human gene to chromosome band 21q22.1, and linkage studies with NIDDM. Diabetes 44: 592-6.

Yamaki A, Noda S, Kudoh J, Shindoh N, Maeda H, Minoshima S, Kawasaki K, Shimizu Y, Shimizu N (1996) The mammalian single-minded (SIM) gene: mouse cDNA structure and diencephalic expression indicate a candidate gene for Down syndrome. Genomics 35: 136-43.

Yaspo ML, Gellen L, Mott R, Korn B, Nizetic D, Poustka AM, Lehrach H (1995) Model for a transcript map of human chromosome 21: isolation of new coding sequences from exon and enriched cDNA libraries. Human Molecular Genetics 4: 1291-1304.

Chapter 19
The Future of Biological Research on Down Syndrome

CHARLES J EPSTEIN

The Goals and Questions

If we think about the future of research on Down syndrome, the major question is the following.

What do we want to achieve?

I would like to suggest that there are several different goals that we would like to accomplish, hopefully in the near future, but certainly over the next decade or two (Table 19.1).

Goal number 1: Probably most important is the prevention or reduction in the frequency of non disjunction leading to trisomy 21. We can work as hard as we want to try to 'cure' the condition and to relieve its symptoms, but ultimately what we would like to be able to do is to prevent Down syndrome from occurring in the first place.

Goal number 2: Since people will continue to be born with Down syndrome no matter what we do, we want to be able to prevent the medical complications of Down syndrome. Although there are many other complications to be considered, the three perhaps most obvious ones are thyroid autoimmunity, infection, and leukemia. Hypothyroidism, which is presumably caused by thyroid autoimmunity, turns out to be a relatively frequent problem. Infection, which in years gone by was a very severe problem, is not such a problem now from the clinical point of view but is still a major contributor to hearing loss, and in the long term, to mortality in Down syndrome. And leukemia, which is not a great problem in quantitative terms, is nonetheless a significant problem when it occurs, and we would certainly like to be able to prevent it.

Goal number 3: We would like to be able to prevent the central nervous system deficits from occurring. Of these, the most important are the deficits in cognition, with difficulties in learning, memory, and thought processes in general, which collectively we call mental retardation.

Although these deficits can be quite variable in extent among individuals with Down syndrome, they nevertheless constitute a pervasive problem. Further, we would like to be able to prevent or ameliorate the difficulties with speech and language which are so frequent in Down syndrome. I have separated speech and language from cognition because people with Down syndrome seem to have a particularly difficult problem in these areas. For example, comparisons between Williams' syndrome and Down syndrome have shown that there are great differences between these two syndromes in cognitive function and speech and language. In Down syndrome, both the formulation and the quality of the speech have created particular difficulties which are superimposed on the cognitive deficits.

Table 19.1 What do we want to achieve?

Prevention or reduction in the frequency of nondisjunction leading to trisomy 21
Prevention of the medical complications of Down syndrome
Thyroid autoimmunity
Infection
Leukemia
Prevention of central nervous system deficits
Cognition
Speech and language
Hypotonia
Prevention of Alzheimer disease
Prevention of the birth of infants with Down syndrome

One other nervous system problem in Down syndrome is hypotonia. It is certainly a problem in the very young infants, and we assume that it also plays some role in the delay in achieving the motor milestones. It also contributes to the cervical problems that we are always concerned about, and we would like to have ways of preventing atlantoaxial instability from occurring. We probably cannot prevent hypotonia since it is present from the time of birth, but the other problems are things that we certainly would like to be able to prevent.

Goal number 4: We would like to prevent the occurrence of Alzheimer disease. We now know that Alzheimer disease, as defined pathologically, occurs in the brains of all persons with Down syndrome by the end of the fourth decade. However, there is still a debate over the proportion of adults with Down syndrome who will ultimately develop the dementia that we associate with Alzheimer disease. Nevertheless, to whatever extent persons with Down syndrome develop dementia, we would like to be able to prevent it from occurring. We are not really worried about the pathology that we cannot see. What we are really worried about are the manifestations of the pathology in terms of its effects on the function of the nervous system and the development of dementia.

Goal number 5: We would like to think about the prevention of the birth of infants with Down syndrome. This brings us to the area of prenatal screening and diagnosis, which must be considered as part of the overall approach to Down syndrome.

Now that we have outlined what we would like to achieve, the next two questions are the following:

Are these goals achievable? If so, how do we go about achieving them?

The prevention or reduction of nondisjunction (Table 19.2)

What do we know about nondisjunction leading to trisomy 21? We know that there is a high frequency of aneuploidy of all types associated with human conception. Indeed, trisomy 21 is not the most frequent form of aneuploidy recognized during gestation. There are other forms that are much more frequent. The remarkable thing is how high the frequency of aneuploidy following human conception actually is. The general thinking is that roughly 15 per cent of known conceptions are spontaneously aborted and that half of these are chromosomally abnormal, and these are just the recognized ones. If we go earlier in gestation and look at conceptions that never last more than a couple of weeks, the frequency of aneuploidy becomes much higher. This is a very important fact which we have to keep in mind as we think about the prevention of nondisjunction. No predisposing factors, either intrinsic or environmental, have been recognized except for maternal age. There has been a suggestion that there may be an influence of the apolipoprotein E genotype, and potentially of other genotypes as well, on the occurrence of nondisjunction. If true, this would be a very important clue to the pathogenesis of nondisjunction. However, for the most part, despite an enormous amount of work looking at all types

Table 19.2 What we know about nondisjunction leading to Trisomy 21

1. There is a high frequency of aneuploidy associated with human conception.

2. There appears to be something inherent in human reproduction which, despite evolution (which ought to favour greater reproductive fitness) has permitted aneuploidy to remain at a high level.

3. No predisposing factors (intrinsic or environmental) have been recognized except for maternal age.

4. Reducing the age of childbearing has the greatest impact on the incidence of trisomy 21.

5. The nature and causes of the maternal age effect are logical points of attack.

6. Chiasma formation and recombination appear to be altered.

7. This is the most specific observation yet and calls for research on the mechanism and regulation of meiosis - human and other.

of environmental factors, only maternal age has consistently been found to be the major factor predisposing to nondisjunction.

As I mentioned earlier, there seems to be something inherent in human reproduction that causes or allows the rate of nondisjunction to remain at a high level. If you try to think about this from the evolutionary point of view, you might think, since such a high rate of spontaneous abortions resulting from aneuploidy would reduce fitness and, thereby, the ability of the species to reproduce, that somehow we should have evolved to the point that we would have reduced this rate if it were at all possible or appropriate to do so. And yet, even though human reproduction is very efficient from the point of view of the fidelity of chromosome replication, the process of chromosome separation does not work so well even after evolution has presumably tried to fine tune it as best as it can. It is this that makes me somewhat pessimistic about being able to attack the problem of nondisjunction in a way that will lead to its reduction or prevention. However, the maternal age effect still remains a logical point of attack in terms of trying to understand the nature of the process that gives rise to nondisjunction. Further implicit in the maternal age effect is the fact that the age at which mothers are having children is the one single alterable factor that influences the frequency of births with trisomy 21. It has been recognized by demographers that as maternal ages shift up and down in the population as a function of various social factors: schooling, jobs, income, when people decide to get married, how many children they decide to have, and many others, the rate of trisomy 21 also rises and falls. Therefore, the quickest way to reduce the frequency of trisomy 21 and Down syndrome would be for everyone to have their children very early (in their early 20s). It does not seem likely that we shall see that. On the contrary, we are now seeing many people waiting until their late 30s to have children. If this trend were not counterbalanced by the expanded use of prenatal diagnosis at this time, the frequency of Down syndrome would be increasing significantly.

It has recently been found that the formation of chiasmata and recombination appear to be altered in the meioses leading to trisomy 21 and Down syndrome, and this is certainly a very important observation. In trisomies in which there is an error in meiosis I, which is the situation in most cases of trisomy 21 that we see, it has been found that the frequency of recombination is much *reduced*. On the other hand, a new finding that has excited people in this field is that with errors occurring in the second meiotic division (meiosis II) there also is an abnormality in the frequency of recombination, but in this case the frequency is much *higher* than normal, especially in the proximal part of the chromosome. These observations that the rate of formation of chiasmata and recombination is altered are the most specific findings that have been made with regard to nondisjunction leading to trisomy 21, and I believe that they justify and call for expanded research on the mechanisms of meiosis, both in humans and in other species. Human meiosis, of course, is very difficult to study, especially in females. Meiosis in other mammals has not been extensively studied, although there is certainly a great deal of work on meiosis in lower organisms of various types, particularly in *Drosophila*. If one takes the point of view that there is likely to be a commonality in the mechanism of meiosis across the many eons of evolution, then much more intensive study on meiotic processes in many organisms is certainly required. And then we are faced with the following question: *Once we find out the mechanisms that are involved in the generation of aneuploidy, will we be able to intervene?*

I'll give you my answer to that at the end of this chapter.

The prevention of the birth of infants with trisomy 21 (Table 19.3)

As was noted earlier, this is essentially the issue of prenatal diagnosis. Prenatal diagnosis has been with us now for roughly 30 years, since the first diagnostic amniocenteses were done to obtain foetal cells for chromosome analysis. Its utilization is still far from complete. A few years ago the figures in the United States indicated that approximately 50 per cent of women over 35 underwent prenatal diagnosis. The figure is probably a little bit higher now, but I suspect that it is not much higher than that and that utilization by women under 35 in terms of either amniocentesis or chorionic villus sampling is very low.

What are the challenges in the area of prenatal diagnosis? I would suggest that there are three. One is the search for earlier and more specific and sensitive markers for the screening of pregnancies. Over the past several years there has been the development of methods for screening all pregnant women to find those who appear to be at a higher risk of carrying a foetus with trisomy 21 or with other chromosome abnormalities. This involves determination of the levels of certain substances in the maternal serum: alphafoetoprotein (AFP), which was the first that was screened for and which tends to run low in trisomy 21 pregnancies, oestriol, and chorionic gonadotropin (HCG). Depending on the specific screening programme, two or three of these markers are usually combined in a way that allows an estimate to be given of the probability of having a trisomic foetus irrespective of the mother's age. The strategy is to screen all pregnant women and then to try to identify those who seem to be at an increased risk. An arbitrary cut off, with a calculated risk of having a child with Down syndrome of the order of about 1 in 300 or greater, is generally used to decide who should go on for further study, such as

Table 19.3 Where is research on the prenatal detection of trisomy 21 leading?

Search for earlier and more specific and sensitive markers for pregnancy screening.
Isolation and analysis of foetal blood cells from the maternal circulation.
Screening by foetal visualization.

amniocentesis. It is important to realize that this is a screening strategy, not a diagnostic one. Presumably it could be extended to more people. It is capable of automation, and it is relatively inexpensive as compared with trying to increase the number of amniocenteses and other diagnostic procedures. However, although maternal serum screening is being used more and more, it certainly is not being offered to all pregnant women, and, even if it were, a significant proportion of cases of Down syndrome would still be missed with this type of screening programme.

Another area in which there is considerable interest now is in the isolation and analysis of foetal blood cells from the maternal circulation. The idea behind this approach relies upon the fact that foetal blood cells go across the placenta and enter the mother's circulation. Therefore, if you had a way of sorting these foetal cells out using, for example, surface markers on the foetal cells that differ from those on the maternal cells, and could look at their chromosomes or at their DNA with techniques other than direct chromosome analysis, you might be able to find which pregnancies are carrying not only trisomy 21 but also a variety of other chromosome abnormalities. This area has been under investigation for a long time, and there are now beginning to appear reports of some successes. Unlike maternal serum screening, foetal cell analysis would be more of a diagnostic than a screening method. However, it would be quite a costly method as now being carried out, although potentially the cost could be reduced. The trick is to be able to isolate the foetal cells which may be present at a frequency of 1 in 10,000 or 1 in 100,000, or even 1 in a million in the maternal circulation, and this is quite a formidable job.

Another approach that was suggested a long time ago, when X-rays were used for diagnosing children with Down syndrome, but is now exciting considerable interest, is the use of foetal visualization. This time it is by ultrasonography, to screen pregnancies for Down syndrome by looking for cystic hygromas or oedema around the neck or at the length of various bones. In very good hands this could be effective screening method, much more sensitive than serum screening and less invasive than amniocentesis or chorionic villus sampling. In fact, with a claimed 80 per cent detection rate at 10-14 weeks of pregnancy, it is close to being diagnostic. However, it requires highly trained ultrasonographers and the appropriate equipment and would not, therefore, be applicable to widescale population screening/diagnosis.

With regard to any approach to the prevention of the birth of children with Down syndrome, the goal would be for detection of affected foetuses to be earlier, more complete, and less invasive.

Prevention of medical complications, central nervous system defects, and Alzheimer disease

The next three items in Table 19.1 will be grouped together because the methodological approaches to arriving at prevention, treatment, and cure are essentially the same. I have tried to conceptualize the approach in the following manner (Figure 19.1). We can start with the phenotypic abnormalities that we see, with the syndrome itself (Figure 19.1, top). Or, we can start with the genes on chromosome 21 (Figure 19.1, bottom). Similarly, we can carry out basic research on common biological mechanisms and processes and on medical disease in general (Figure 19.1, left), or we can carry out clinical research looking at particular phenotypic abnormalities (Figure 19.1, right).

I have separated out this 'side by side' approach of going from either the basic research or the clinical research side, either of which may not necessarily be research aimed at Down syndrome itself, from the 'top and bottom' approaches in Figure 19.1 to make the following point. Much of what happens in medicine with regard to any specific disease or condition does not necessarily come about by targeted research. Rather, it may result from discoveries made during the course of research being carried for entirely different reasons and on quite different problems which, all of a sudden, become quite relevant to the issue with which you are concerned. So, if we think about Down syndrome and the different aspects of the phenotype that we are interested in, basic and clinical research in neuroscience and on neurologic processes, on how the brain and immune system work, on the development of malignancy and so on are likely to have real benefits for the Down syndrome situation. Accordingly, I think that we have to take a broader view than just to think that only work that is directly targeted to Down syndrome is what

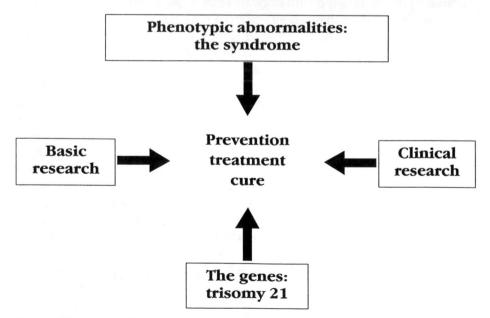

Figure 19.1 Methodological approaches to prevention, treatment and cure.

is going to end up helping people with Down syndrome. Research that is being done in a whole variety of areas is also likely to help. For example, there is an enormous amount of work being done in the field of Alzheimer disease, not because most people with Down syndrome develop Alzheimer disease but because most of the members of the general population will, if they live long enough, get some form of dementia. Therefore, research on Alzheimer disease is likely to have tremendous ramifications for Down syndrome, as will Down syndrome for Alzheimer disease research. From the Down syndrome point of view, I think that we can just sit back and look at what is happening in the Alzheimer disease field and say, 'Well, sooner or later they will find things that will help our people as well'.

If we think about research on the phenotypic abnormalities of Down syndrome, a sort of a 'top-down' approach, this is the approach that has been used for the last 100 years. Although it might be thought that we have exhausted the top-down approach, I suggest that we not only have not exhausted it, we really have not even begun to work on the tougher problems. For example, we need to have an improved definition of the specific and characteristic deficits of cognition, language and of other aspects of nervous system function in Down syndrome and of the neuro-physiological, neurochemical, neuroanatomical alterations that cause them. We cannot do this in the mouse, we cannot do it in the monkey, and we certainly cannot do it in the fruit fly. What we somehow have to figure out is how to do it with people with Down syndrome. We have to try to understand, in much more precise and specific terms than have been used thus far, what the problems in cognition are, where the deficits in language come from, what other aspects of the nervous system are not functioning well. Although we have lots of clues, we just have not been able to put them together. For example, although it has been known for many years that the evoked electrical responses to various stimuli are abnormal, I have yet to see a really good explanation of what is wrong in transmitting the message from the ear or the eye to the cortex. Clearly, we need to get into these aspects of the phenotype to be able to move forward.

Much of current research on Down syndrome is concerned with what we might call the 'bottom-up' approach, starting with chromosome 21 and then working toward the phenotype. This involves the mapping, cloning, sequencing, and delineation of the functions of the genes on chromosome 21 and then determining the consequences of their overexpression. To do this kind of work, the genomics approach is certainly important, and it appears, if everyone's predictions are correct, that in the next several years chromosome 21 will be sequenced and the genes identified. And then we will start a very long process involving biochemistry, physiology, and cell biology with a variety of systems to determine just what all these genes are doing and why having increased numbers of them causes problems.

Assumptions underlying the genetic approach

When we take a 'bottom-up' genetic approach to try to understand the pathogenesis of Down syndrome, there are certain implicit assumptions that we make.

Assumption number 1: If we are going to go to all of the trouble of identifying the genes on chromosome 21 and to figure out what they are doing, we must assume is that the phenotype of Down syndrome results from the increased number of copies of the genes present on chromosome 21 and not from some non-specific effects of chromosome imbalance. This may seem to be an almost trivial assumption, but even to this day there are some who question it. The argument supporting it is fairly straightforward: As a pattern of phenotypic components, Down syndrome looks like Down syndrome and does not look like any of the other 150 or 200 clinical trisomies that we know about.

Assumption number 2: We are not going to find one gene that causes the entire phenotype of Down syndrome. This may appear to be a silly thing to have to say, but there still is, in the minds of many people and in the literature, the expectation that there is or will be 'the gene that causes Down syndrome'. There is no such single gene, in my view, that causes all of Down syndrome. There are many genes that give rise to Down syndrome. So, to take the approach that there is one gene is, I am afraid, going to lead to futility.

Assumption number 3: Specific components of the phenotype of Down syndrome can be attributed to the imbalance of individual genes (Figure 19.2). This does not mean that each feature results from imbalance of a different gene or of only a single gene, although it may be true to a limited extent for certain things. It might be true for leukemia and for duodenal stenosis and maybe even for heart disease. But, I think it is likely not to be true for very many things, and it is certainly not likely to be true for the central nervous system. So we have to make a few modifying assumptions: some or many genes on chromosome 21 may contribute to a particular component of the phenotype; conversely, some or perhaps many of the components of the phenotype may result from the interactions or independent actions of two or more chromosome 21 genes which do not have to be contiguous with one another and may be extremely difficult to identify in the human situation. It is for this reason that animal models for Down syndrome are being developed and studied. We have ways by which we can make the trisomies in the mouse and of manipulating the mouse genome to determine which genes are contributing to some component of the phenotype.

A related issue which poses a very difficult problem is that there is no a priori way to determine the number of genes involved in the genesis of a complex phenotype such as we have in Down syndrome. We don't really know, when we start, how many genes we want to look for. Although methods which make use of family studies are being developed for other complex disorders such as diabetes and atherosclerosis, it s unlikely that they will be applicable to Down syndrome.

If we consider Figure 19.2 in more detail, it illustrates what we are likely to find as we study the genetic basis of Down syndrome. There will be genes that will affect several different components of the phenotype, some of which may be caused by imbalance of single gene. Some components of the phenotype will be produced by imbalance of more than one chromosome 21 gene. In addition, there may be contributions from genes not on chromosome 21, which are represented by the dashed line in Figure 19.2, to the development of particular components of the phenotype. Chromosome 21 is only one of the 22 sets of autosomcs in the human genome, in addition to the sex chromosome. Since genes do not function in isolation, whatever the genes on chromosome 21 are doing will be influenced by genes on other chromosomes. These genes, as well as the genes on chromosome 21 itself, may differ in subtle ways from one person to another. We use the term 'polymorphic' to refer to genes which may have one or more variants which differ from each other in minor ways which, nevertheless, may affect their functions. The likely influence of such polymorphic genes is of importance when we consider the phenotype of Down syndrome. Although people with Down syndrome are recognizably similar to one another in the overall pattern of physical features and functional deficits that collectively define the syndrome, when you look at persons with Down syndrome in fine detail, each one is very different from the others. Therefore, whereas the actions of the genes on chromosome 21 are powerful enough, when present in three copies, for us to recognize that the syndrome in present, there is enough variability in how the syndrome manifests to tell us that we have to keep in mind how all the rest of the genome is interacting and influencing the development of the syndrome.

COMPONENTS OF PHENOTYPE

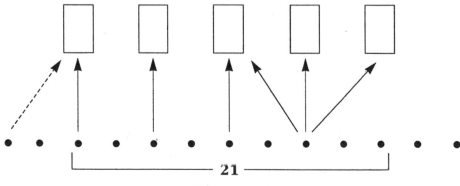

The genes

Figure 19.2 Specific components of the phenotype of Down syndrome

When it comes to the issue of cognitive deficits or mental retardation, I do not think the imbalance of a single gene will be found to be responsible for all the cognitive and language deficits in Down syndrome. Many chromosome 21 genes are expressed in the nervous system, each of which can be considered to be an interesting gene and potentially very important for the development of mental retardation. In fact, they all might be important, and it is for this reason that I do not think that any one of them is going to be 'the' gene for mental retardation. There are likely to be several. Furthermore, there are many different components to the retardation and cognitive deficits in Down syndrome, and, as I mentioned earlier, these deficits are not the same for all retarded persons or even all persons with Down syndrome. Hopefully we will find that there are some genes that play a more major role than do others. Some of these genes may affect just one aspect of the retardation and some may affect several, but ultimately these will have to be teased apart.

I regard the identification of the major genes contributing to the cognitive and speech and language deficits in Down syndrome to be a very formidable problem from the genetic point of view, given our inability to carry out the relevant genetic experiments in the human situation. Therefore, do we need to consider the extent to which trisomic animals can be used as models for the cognitive deficits in Down syndrome? This is a question that most of us who work in the field of animal models for Down syndrome think about all the time. After all, a mouse is a mouse and a human is a human, and we cannot assume that mouse behaviour necessarily models human behaviour. Nevertheless, to the extent that we can fractionate the behavioural and learning deficits which we find in the experimental animals, we might be able to find out which genes have the major effects on the abnormal functioning of the central nervous system in the Down syndrome models.

The Future

So, given all that I have said, how do I view the future of research on Down syndrome?

With guarded optimism.

I think important things are going to happen and that a tremendous amount of progress is going to occur, but I do not want to promise more than is likely to be delivered. Here, then, are my predictions.

Prediction number 1: The causative mechanisms in the genesis of aneuploidy are likely to be better understood, but a reduction in the rate of nondisjunction leading to trisomy 21 is less likely to be achieved. Frankly, I am fairly pessimistic about really being able to drive down the rate of nondisjunction. It does not mean we should not try. I think that it is a most worthy goal, but I just have the 'gut' feeling that we do not understand the reason why frequency of aneuploidy is as high as it is and that we are not going to be able to reduce it without changing something else that may cause us more difficulty than we can anticipate.

Prediction number 2: There will be more complete but probably not total identification of pregnancies carrying a foetus with trisomy 21. There will certainly not be total identification from the social point of view in terms of the population at large because of the relative scarcity of resources. But, even if resources were not an issue, it must be realized that not every woman wants to have her pregnancy tested and a trisomic foetus identified. There is a significant proportion of people who do not wish to interfere with the pregnancy, whatever the outcome. So, no matter how far we are able to go, we are certainly not going to eliminate the birth of children with trisomy 21 or other chromosomal problems because people are just not going to allow that to occur.

Prediction number 3: Human chromosome 21 will be completely mapped and sequenced, the expressed genes will be identified, their functions will be defined. The last of these, the definition of functions, will take the most time.

Prediction number 4: The gene or genes responsible for many components of the Down syndrome phenotype, including heart disease, duodenal atresia/stenosis, inmunological impairment, leukemia and Alzheimer disease, will be identified. It may take a long time for some of these, but I think that identification of these genes will ultimately be achievable.

Prediction number 5: Specific and characteristic cognitive deficits that distinguish Down syndrome from other forms of mental retardation will be elucidated, and genes responsible for major deficits in cognition will be discovered. How many of the genes or what fraction of the genes that really play the major role will be discovered, I cannot really say.

Prediction number 6: There is a good likelihood of developing pharmacological and other forms of therapy that will ameliorate - and perhaps even prevent - mental retardation and Alzheimer disease. I make this prediction separate from any considerations concerning genes and other things because I believe that there is an enormous amount of progress which is occurring in neuroscience and neuropharmacology that has absolutely nothing to do with Down syndrome but has a great deal to do with how the nervous system works. This knowledge should ultimately work to the benefit of people with Down syndrome.

Final prediction and conclusion

Prediction number 7: It is probably not essential that we know all of the genes on chromosome 21 before rational therapies can be considered. As we continue to learn more about how the brain works, research on Down syndrome will ultimately be the beneficiary of this knowledge and an understanding of what is impairing the function of the brain will ultimately be attained. With this understanding will come the approaches required for preventing or correcting the situation.

With regard to therapies, the operative word is *rational*!

So, as I said earlier, I am guardedly optimistic that a great deal of progress will be made in understanding Down syndrome and that we will come closer to achieving our goals of preventing, treating, and curing it. This progress will come from all sides: from the genetic and phenotypic approaches, from basic science and clinical research. All will be of importance.

Acknowledgement

The author's work on Down syndrome has been supported by NIH grants HD 31498 and AG 08938.

PART 7
DOWN SYNDROME IN THE WORLD

Chapter 20
The World Association Movement for Down Syndrome

JUAN PERERA

Keys of the World Association Movement for Down Syndrome

The history of the world association movement for Down syndrome during the last decade of the twentieth century shows that the aim has been to consolidate the common strength of this independent movement in the world's developed countries, seeking public commitment and collaboration, claiming the representative nature of the collective and organizing more solid and better managed structures. Families, professionals and persons with Down syndrome, *working together* in the associations and federations, have tried to adapt to the circumstances, to contribute new and specific solutions, to change social attitudes and respond efficiently to the needs of persons with Down syndrome, which is *basically the only thing that should really matter to us*.

Is it possible for us to talk about a philosophy of our association movement? Do we share a set of ideas and good practices that the majority of the world organizations for persons with Down syndrome assume and accept? Are we clear about the paths we should take as we approach the twenty-first century?

To answer these questions, I would like to submit for the consideration of the congress delegates and leaders of the world association movement for Down syndrome, some suggestions and ideas that I have summarized after a close study of the statutes and declarations of more than 40 active associations for Down syndrome from all over the world.

Philosophy of the World Association Movement for Down Syndrome: Basic Principles

1. The principle that the capabilities of persons with Down's syndrome should take precedence over their limitations or differences is assumed

from the affirmation of human dignity in which such persons are included.

2. As a result of the Universal Declaration of Human Rights, United Nations' documents and the World Action Programme for Disabled People, it is affirmed that 'the principle of equal rights' between people with and without a disability means that the needs of all individuals have the same importance, that these needs have to form the basis for social planning and that all resources have to be used in such a way that they guarantee equal opportunities for everyone.

3. Our association movement defends the stance that equal rights in health, education, work, social services, culture and leisure are only possible by using ordinary community services, which have to respond to the needs of people with Down syndrome to the same standard as apply to the rest of the population.

4. It is affirmed that personalized and specialized attention in prevention, health, education, employment and similar programmes will tend to cover the specific needs of people with Down syndrome and will be applied by specialists in ordinary centres or services.

5. Normalization and inclusion at all levels and in all services are defended and only exceptionally, when integration is not possible because of the severity or complexity of the limitations presented by the person with Down syndrome, will that person be attended to in special services or centres, with the family's agreement.

6. It is obvious that special attention is given to the quality of life for people with Down syndrome; this being understood as a) that their needs and expectations are covered; b) that they develop their potentialities; and c) that they enjoy all their rights. Almost all associations refer in one way or another to the term 'quality of life'.

7. The fight for equality is proposed from the point of view of solidarity, but with respect for diversity in an open and plural society enriched by this diversity and with the active participation of people with Down syndrome.

8. Association leadership is understood from the point of view of tolerance to be a respectful form of collaborating and participating with all the legally constituted organizations which respect the rights of disabled people, without wishing to resort to competition or confrontation under any circumstances. That is to say, conserving its own identity.

These principles, drawn as I have said from the statutes and declarations of many associations for Down syndrome from all over the world, if placed in logical order could very well constitute a good universal declaration of the principles of the world association movement for Down syndrome.

However, if principles and ideas are important, so too are good practices. In this case it is much more difficult to try to summarize what is being done in the most active associations in the world because a wide range of variables are involved: standard of development, social habits, customs, ethical principles, government collaboration, and so on.

Good Practices

We can, however, try to state some commonly accepted good practices.

Starting from the principle that everyone with Down syndrome has the right to receive the personalized and specialized attention they need, the mission of our associations is to:

- detect these needs;
- transmit them to the relevant public organizations
- collaborate in solving them; and in two ways:
  a) demanding from the relevant public organizations an efficient and suitable response from the community's ordinary services;
  b) establishing and rendering the necessary services when the public organizations do not have them. In this case, quality services have to be offered; they have to be addressed in the same way as companies rendering services to customers (the customer concept implies the right to demand); they have to come under the criteria of a nonprofitmaking economy (audits, inspection, and so on).

Priorities

It is not easy to catalogue our associations' objectives and priorities. Nevertheless, with great respect for what is being done elsewhere and while emphasizing not only that there is not one single method, system or way, but also that what works in one place probably does not work everywhere, I would like to present to you, even though it is in the form of a list, the priorities that our associations establish in their programmes:

In our priorities most emphasis is put on the specificity of the world association movement for Down syndrome, which at the same time is the greatest difference between our movement and the associations attending to the psychologically disabled in general.

1. Prevention. Early diagnosis and genetic advice. It is obvious that good information helps parents to make more responsible decisions and be better prepared to accept their children with Down syndrome.
2. Defence of rights. The associations for Down syndrome will ensure the defence of equal rights recognized by international law for all citizens and will strongly denounce any violations.
3. Specialists' training. The complete training of professionals (physicians, psychologists, educators, speech therapists, trainers for employment, physiotherapists, and so on) is fundamental for people with

Down syndrome to obtain specialized medical and educational attention in the community's ordinary services in accordance with their needs.

4. Health programmes. Good health is the basis for intellectual development, as well as for a better quality of life and longer life expectancy. Specific medical problems have to be diagnosed and resolved as soon as possible.

5. Early care programmes. It has been demonstrated that owing to the brain's plasticity during the first years of life early, specific and well-applied care programmes are efficient because the children who have followed them improve their cognitive and adaptation capacities.

6. The school of diversity. School has to supply the answer to the educational needs of all its pupils, whether they have a disability or not. No effort must be spared to supply schools, public and private ones, with the necessary supports and resources, including those of teacher training, and for curriculum adaptations to be a fact.

7. Support for inclusion in school. Children and young people with Down syndrome who are of school age and are ready to be integrated in ordinary school and yet have not received sufficient specialized support from the relevant education authority will be subject to special attention.

8. Employment. Professional training must prepare for work and for life. The government must give priority to creating jobs in the ordinary labour framework because work means having greater autonomy and being recognized as an adult before the family and before society.

9. Support for the families. From the very beginning the family, as the first natural nucleus of integration for the person with Down syndrome, must have the correct information and proper training, leading to full acceptance of the situation and to effective involvement in the care and education. Likewise, the family must be given support services and rest.

10. Care for the seriously disabled. There are people with Down syndrome who have a profound psychological or physical disability, whose chances of recovery, adaptation to the environment and integration in society are very limited and who constitute a heavy burden for their families. They will receive care, as soon as each case and its special characteristics have been studied, in highly specialized centres, ensuring that the best possible standard of normalization is achieved in each particular situation.

11. Recognizing the role of the adult and self-advocacy. An education in accordance with the principles of normalization and integration which is based on the potentialities of the individual leads to a higher level of autonomy and to adopting the adult role. This implies the right to self-advocacy and facilitates integration in work, a relationship with a partner, an independent life and is the best guarantee for facing old age alone.

12. Bringing the services closer to the users. The services must be brought closer to users so that attention can be given to the specific needs in each place.
13. Sensitization, image and promotion. The associations will ensure that a positive image of the person with Down syndrome is promoted in society, from the perspective that diversity enriches the whole.
14. Support for research and the implantation of new technologies. New scientific applications in health care and in the general attention given to the person with Down syndrome will be the object of constant concern so that there is a permanent adaptation of services to scientific standards.
15. Guardianship services. By supporting the creation of Guardianship Foundations disabled people are guaranteed to receive correct attention when the family cannot attend to them.
16. Leisure services and free time. To improve the social integration, personal autonomy and enjoyment of recreational activities of people with Down syndrome.

Future Prospects

You are aware of the enormous strength and energy of our associations, but the different challenges we are facing have to be put clearly in focus if we want them to have future prospects. What are these challenges?

1. The first of these could be *effectiveness*. I believe that our associations have to think about achieving results. Good intentions are not enough. We have to achieve what we propose. If our mission is to improve the quality of life of people with Down syndrome, we must evaluate the results. If we propose modifying certain social or political criteria, we have to be effective and achieve maximum collaboration from society.

   This approach to effectiveness has to lead to a reassessment of our organization, our operation and our training. The mission, what we propose to do, is the most important thing, not the entity, nor the persons, nor the professionals, who are only the means; an instrument at the service of a cause.

2. The second challenge is that of *specificity* or *specialization*. Nobody today denies the specificity of Down syndrome. There are numerous publications all over the world emphasizing the unique and particular aspects of Down syndrome which do not occur in other kinds of mental retardation (or which occur in a different proportion) and which therefore mark the limits with other kinds of cerebral pathology. The molecular structure of chromosome 21 shows a series of genetic anomalies which, in turn, cause a series of disorders in the brain and in the nervous system for the entire life of people with Down syndrome and which condition their learning and conduct. The more we know

about these specific aspects, the better we will be able to design therapeutic methods and educational strategies that will prove to be more
direct and effective for their rehabilitation.

3. The third challenge is a direct consequence of the previous one (that of
    specificity), and that is the *independence* of our associations with
    respect to associations attending to psychological disabilities in
    general. Present-day research shows that mental retardation cannot be
    tackled as one single entity, as it embraces distinct and different
    symptoms, both from the neuropathological and neuropsychological
    points of view. The associations of a general nature have not provided
    the right answer to the needs of people with Down syndrome. That is
    why families have sought more progressive and up-to-date solutions
    through the associations for Down syndrome. There is also another
    important reason, and that is the high number in the collective: there
    are approximately five million people with Down syndrome in the
    world. Is that not a sufficient number for the collective to have its own
    organization and infrastructure without having to depend on anyone
    else? Let it be made quite clear - as I have said before: independence
    does not mean confrontation, neither does it mean denying the many
    things that are shared in common with the associations working for
    people with mental retardation nor denying collaboration on certain
    matters.

4. The fourth challenge is that of *coordination of effort*. All too often
    problems arise in the associations between the parents and profes-
    sionals, between the associations and centres or services on which
    these depend, between official and private interests. Our associations
    have to make sure that they are above personal interests, professional
    conflicts, political or religious ideas or any stumbling-block separating
    them from the only thing that really matters: working to improve the
    quality of life for people with Down syndrome. One cannot, nor
    should one, disregard anyone. The coordination of efforts for a
    common objective will be achieved if parents, professionals and the
    people with Down syndrome themselves work together, putting aside
    personal considerations and struggles for power.

5. The fifth challenge is *consolidation*. Our local associations, regional or
    national federations and our international confederations need to be
    stabilized internally in order to acquire the character of democratic
    change. Too frequently the same persons head an organization for ten
    or more years. This is not good. The 'personal' work - extraordinary at
    times - ends with the person, and then comes the disaster. We are all
    necessary, but no one should think that they are indispensable.
    Organizations should ensure their stability and their continuity with
    turns being taken in office: sometimes the parents, at other times the
    professionals, whoever is better able to do it in each case, and always
    counting on the actual people with Down syndrome who, more and

more, are taking a leading role and want to be their own protectors and defenders.

6. The sixth challenge is *collaboration*. The associations for Down syndrome cannot isolate themselves. The complexity of society today demands the combined intervention of various kinds of entities. While conserving our identity, we have to be capable of seeking and finding spaces for collaboration with other associations who are working with the same aims. We have to find the points that unite us rather than those that separate us. United we can do more and better things. Collaboration and coordination with associations in the sector is - in my opinion - a moral obligation which has to serve to overcome the present mini-nature of the associations. *We have to be happy about the triumphs of others*, such as when someone brings out a new publication, achieves resources for research or attains greater social recognition.

   This collaboration has to be extended towards government administration. We should not regard each other as enemies, but as collaborators. We have to ensure that confrontation or servility are not the only means possible for a relationship. We have to take steps towards agreements: our associations cooperate with government administration in providing certain services and in some way we are substituting for them by offering services which they should be giving. Probably we do it better and at a lower cost. However, it is necessary to ensure agreements that are over and above political changes and specific individuals.

7. The seventh challenge is that of *transparency*. If the associations for Down syndrome want the support of people and organizations, administrations, companies and the media, we have to make an effort to be transparent.

   This means transparent in our ideologies and approaches. Transparent in our message and intentions. Transparent in our organizations, in our 'dependencies', connections or obligations. Above all, transparent in the forms of financing and economic management. Transparency is, in this case, synonymous with trust and credibility. We have to avoid the obscure. We have to banish doubt. This is important when public funds are involved, but it is even more so when the funds proceed from solidarity.

8. I would like to give a rather provocative name to the eighth and last challenge: *disobedience*. With this term I would like to refer to the need that our associations have to dedicate time, reflection and efforts to constructing what we could call the particular 'culture' of our association movement in the world.

   I believe that future prospects will be determined - to a great extent - by the capacity we have to get to the heart of those elements that most obviously and clearly identify us. In the theoretical aspects (philosophical-conceptual) as well as in the most practical aspects (strategies, organization, operation). Our hallmark is based on *the rights that people with Down syndrome have* to be treated without any discrimination, in a society that is enriched by diversity. Too frequently we accept charity, welfare, exceptions, when our struggle and our 'disobedience' should be claiming constitutional rights that are all too often and in many parts of the world still being denied to persons with Down syndrome.

I know that the challenges I have proposed are difficult. Above all, I know that the challenges in the developing countries are ones of survival and claiming basic rights. However, it seems to me important that we should be clear about the model to follow, the objectives to achieve and that those less advanced societies can count on the unconditional support of the more developed countries.

Let us hope that between us all we are capable of building a better future for people with Down syndrome.

Let us hope that our dreams come true in the twenty-first century when we meet at the next World Congress in the year 2000.

PART 8
CONCLUSIONS

Postscript: Perspectives on Down Syndrome

JEAN A RONDAL, JUAN PERERA AND LYNN NADEL

Looking back on the state of affairs in Down syndrome over the last 40 years, one cannot fail to notice the formidable changes that have occurred. Not so long ago there was ignorance regarding its exact cause, a total lack of adequate care and education for affected babies and children, and societal insensitivity for grown-up persons with Down syndrome.

In the late 1950s, we learned that Down syndrome was a genetic syndrome caused by trisomy 21. In the 1960s, several countries organized open school classes for children with Down syndrome and other conditions conducive to moderate or severe mental retardation. Professionals began to advise raising these babies and children in the family as opposed to the previous practice of institutionalization. In the late 1960s and early 1970s, continuing to the present day, parents and professionals joined efforts in many parts of the world to create specific associations, frequently with little assistance from public services. They urged the scientific community to involve its members in a search for ways to improve the health, development, education, and social welfare of persons affected with Down syndrome. They demanded that the condition of the infant be disclosed and discussed with greater humanity by the medical profession and fought for proper medical treatment of their children. Progressively, the situation improved, at least in the developed countries. Increased medical concern and attention led to healthier Down syndrome babies and children in growing numbers. The application of surgical techniques permitted the saving of many lives. As a result, life expectancy has increased significantly in Down syndrome and infant mortality has been greatly reduced.

From the early 1970s on, psychologists, paediatricians, and educators have teamed up to organize and deliver early intervention programmes intended to stimulate growth, promote development, and better socialize the young child with Down syndrome, in many cases incorporating the families in the early remediation efforts.

The need to encourage school integration for a larger number of children with Down syndrome emerged particularly in the late 1970s and early 1980s. Nonsegregative schooling has come to be considered as a right by a growing number of parents of Down syndrome children.

The further integration of adolescents and adults with Down syndrome into society as responsible citizens then became the next logical step. Though this battle is far from being won, it has absorbed considerable energy since the early 1980s. Lastly, more attention and care is now directed towards adults and ageing persons with Down syndrome, trying to address better the particular psychological and health problems that may complicate the life of these persons as remote consequences of their constitutional pathology.

Thus, progress over the last 40 years has been impressive. The programme of the VI World Congress reflects the extraordinary dynamism of the Down syndrome community at national and international levels as well as the scope and richness of the questions raised and solutions envisaged and worked out in many parts of the world.

So there are good reasons to hope for a better future for persons with Down syndrome and their families. We must keep in mind, however, that the journey is far from over. There remains as much to be done as has already been accomplished, even though it is often true that the early steps are the most difficult.

Persisting challenges for future concern and activities regarding persons with Down syndrome and their families are numerous. Among the most important and urgent ones, one may note the following:

1. increased recognition of the syndromic specificity of Down syndrome;
2. better knowledge of the genetic mechanisms inducing Down syndrome and of the individual variation at the genetic and epigenetic level (particularly brain development);
3. more precise characterization of psychological, educational, and social development in Down syndrome individuals;
4. continued improvement of medical care for the whole lifecycle of Down syndrome individuals;
5. better and specialized school techniques and approaches for tracking literacy and computational skills in Down syndrome children and adolescents;
6. more effective ways of integrating Down syndrome individuals in society and making them feel and be full-fledged members of our social structures;
7. adequate medical, psychological, and social care of ageing Down syndrome persons.

Caring and advanced societies have the privilege of setting high standards for the management and upbringing of their least favoured members. The next World Congress will take place in Sydney, Australia in 2000. Let us hope that the twenty-first century will fulfil our dream of witnessing societies without the unfortunate barriers that have existed for a long time, and with particular force in modern times.

Conclusions of the VI World Congress on Down Syndrome

JEAN A RONDAL, JUAN PERERA AND LYNN NADEL

The aim of the VI Congress was to provide an answer to the challenges facing persons with Down syndrome as the twenty-first century approaches, stressing the following proposals:

1. The promotion of *genetic investigation* in order to probe deeper into chromosome 21's identity (especially finding out which genes are responsible and how they interact), as well as to probe into the mechanisms causing *nondisjunction*, with the aim of preventing or reducing the appearance of the syndrome.
2. The study of *specificity* in Down syndrome, trying to isolate typical characteristics so that it is possible to design more efficient instruments of a medical and psychopedogogical nature for the rehabilitation and education of persons with Down syndrome.
3. The search for *practical solutions* (strategies, programmes, methods, and so on) which, taking into account the findings of recent scientific research, provide concrete solutions applicable to the health care, early attention, education, social and labour integration of persons with Down syndrome.
4. To specify a *quality of life* model for persons with Down syndrome with three particular aspects: a) that their needs and expectations are met; b) that they develop all their potentialities; c) that they enjoy all their rights.
5. In the *area of health*: an endeavour must be made to spread and establish *preventive medical programmes for persons with Down syndrome* everywhere in the world and also to maintain a critical attitude towards therapies not confirmed scientifically. By applying the principle 'the same cases require the same treatment', organ transplants for persons with Down syndrome who require them should be encouraged.
6. Becoming aware of the important role of *the family as the Down syndrome person's first natural nucleus of integration* will encourage actions addressed towards effective training and the involvement of

parents in the, education and social insertion of their children.

7. Specialized attention must preferentially reach *those persons with Down syndrome who have other additional serious limitations or needs* that prevent their effective integration. Attention could be given to them in specialized centres, with the support of the family, attaining the level of normalization that is possible in each case.

8. In the *field of education* the Congress decisively supported three criteria: a) *inclusion*, with the proper supports, in an ordinary school; b) *specific* programmes and curriculum adaptations; c) the application of *new technologies* in the classroom as a particularly useful strategy.

9. The Congress called attention to the importance that *the adult life of persons with Down syndrome* has at the present time, including *self-advocacy*, in such a way that the services provided are adapted to their rights, needs and demands, guaranteeing a positive quality of life.

10. All the means at our disposal must be used to encourage *effective integration* of persons with Down syndrome in school, work, culture and social life, with the understanding that nondiscrimination means equal opportunities. Likewise, the change towards a better social image and participation of persons with Down syndrome in public life must be pursued.

11. Training and *employment* of Down syndrome persons in ordinary firms must be a priority as a source of personal realization and autonomy and full participation in the life of the community.

12. Encouragement must be given to the worldwide creation of *specific associations* for Down syndrome, *independent* from the associations which attend to persons with mental retardation in general. These associations should claim representation and financial support from governmental departments.

13. The Down syndrome *associations* must ensure that *parents, professionals and persons with Down syndrome* are integrated in their organization and management and they must be guided and reorganized by democratic principles.

14. *The services* - to be created whenever necessary - have to respond to criteria of quality, efficiency and social economy and insofar as is possible they have to be *rendered and integrated* in the normal services of the community.

15. The training of specialists in university and in postgraduate courses is fundamental if persons with Down syndrome are to receive global and specialized attention in accordance with their needs.

Mr S Al Malaq (Saudi Arabia), Prof F Astudillo (Spain), Prof M Beeghly (USA), Prof RI Brown (Australia), Prof S Buckley (UK), Prof C Epstein (USA), Prof A Fortuny (Spain), Prof C García Pastor (Spain), Prof MJ Guralnick (USA), Prof R Hodapp (USA), Mrs M Madnick (USA), Mrs J Mills (Canada), Prof E Momotani (Japan), Prof E Montobbio (Italy), Prof F

Murphy (USA), Prof L Nadel (USA), Prof RR Olbrisch (Germany), Prof J Perera (Spain), Prof S Pueschel (USA), Prof A Rasore-Quartino (Italy), Mrs P Robertson (Indonesia), Prof JA Rondal (Belgium), Prof J Rynders (USA), Prof B Sacks (UK), Mrs M Schoeman (South Africa), Prof W Silverman (USA), Prof PM Sinet (France), Mrs R Sneh (Israel), Prof DC Van Dyke (USA), Prof JE Wänn (Sweden), Prof HA Wisniewski (USA), Prof K Wisniewski (USA).

Subject Index